ON THE TRAIL OF THE MORNING STAR

Before you start to read this book, take this moment to think about making a donation to punctum books, an independent non-profit press

@ https://punctumbooks.com/support

If you're reading the e-book, you can click on the image below to go directly to our donations site. Any amount, no matter the size, is appreciated and will help us to keep our ship of fools afloat. Contributions from dedicated readers will also help us to keep our commons open and to cultivate new work that can't find a welcoming port elsewhere. Our adventure is not possible without your support.

Vive la Open Access.

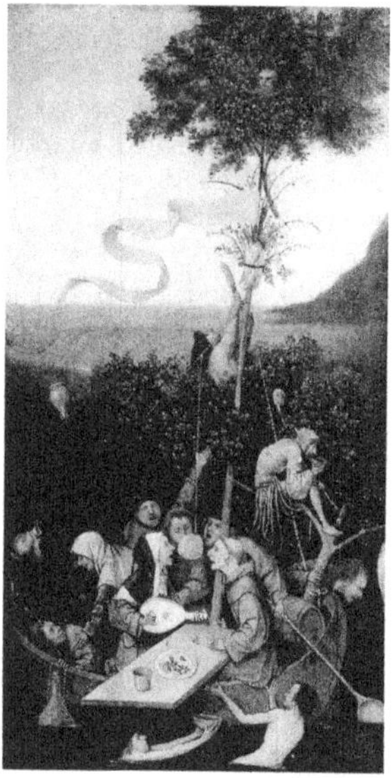

Fig. 1. Detail from Hieronymus Bosch, *Ship of Fools* (1490–1500)

Originally published as Dorothea Buck-Zerchin, *Auf der Spur des Morgensterns: Psychose als Selbstfindung*, ed. Hans Krieger (Neumünster: Paranus Verlag/Norderstedt: Anne Fischer Verlag, 2005).
First English translation published in 2024 by 3Ecologies Books/Immediations, an imprint of punctum books.
https://punctumbooks.com

ISBN-13: 978-1-68571-152-8 (print)
ISBN-13: 978-1-68571-153-5 (ePDF)

DOI: 10.53288/0462.1.00

LCCN: 2024937652
Library of Congress Cataloging Data is available from the Library of Congress

Book design: Hatim Eujayl
Cover design: Vincent W.J. van Gerven Oei
Cover photo: Raphael Schwinger, Wangerooge, 2013.

punctumbooks
spontaneous acts of scholarly combustion

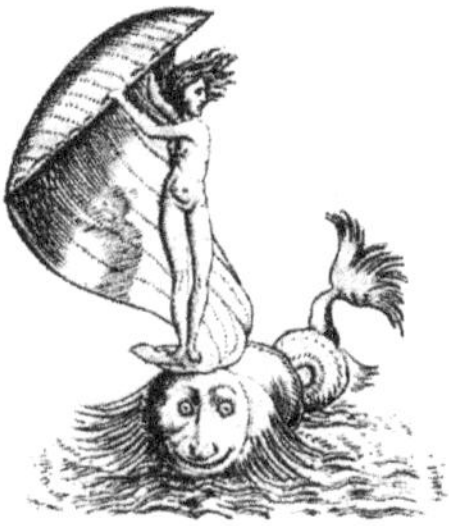

HIC SVNT MONSTRA

3

Dorothea Buck

On the Trail of the Morning Star

Psychosis as Self-Discovery

edited by Susanne Antonetta
translated by Eva Lipton

Contents

Acknowledgments

In the years after my own healing, I wrote many letters to psychiatrists. I wanted them to understand that understanding psychotic experiences is essential to cure schizophrenia; such understanding can come about in group discussions. My efforts were in vain. It seems our psychiatrists worry about their own expertise, when patients are given a voice to speak of their own experience of psychosis and are taken seriously.

Hans Krieger freed me from this silent powerlessness by giving me his interest, his encouragement, and his advice. Without his constructive sympathy over many years, I would not have written this account of my own experiences in psychosis, and my own healing through understanding them.

I also thank my sisters for their encouragement and advice.

Dorothea Buck

Trails

On the English Edition of Dorothea Buck's *On the Trail of the Morning Star: Psychosis as Self-Discovery*

Susanne Paola Antonetta

I first encountered Dorothea Buck in 2019, when I needed her. Buck appeared in many people's lives this way, when needed. This is the way of appearing I think she preferred. Buck died that fall, at the age of one hundred and two, as I was having a psychotic episode. I learned of Buck's life and her book through an obituary in *The New York Times*.

I found her memoir, *On the Trail of the Morning Star*, and had it translated. I encountered a thinker who captured not only the buffeting of psychosis, but its corollary: the mind engaged in a process of world-making, a making that functions through its own channels. Buck did not deny the pain psychosis can cause. She also believed psychotic experience cries out for careful understanding. In that understanding lies growth. Buck taught me a new respect for the wildly creative work of consciousness.

Buck argued throughout her life for a redefinition of psychosis, one that would change the attitudes of the psychosis experiencer and the medical field that labels and defines us. At the age of ninety she addressed a special congress of the World Psychiatric Association and posed this question: "What would be the consequences if it weren't you psychiatrists who had the power of definition, but if the power were ours?" This question is still unanswered. Dorothea Buck has many labels: psychotic, psychiatric victim, Nazi victim, Jungian, activist, reformer, even prophet. All these fit, but none snugly. Her transparence to experience is one of the most remarkable parts of *Morning Star:* the way life, whether hard or easy, moved through her to form a cohesive vision. By the end of the book, she's lived herself into a place as much the province of philosophy as of life history.

Dorothea Buck was born in Naumburg, Germany, in 1917, the fourth of five children. Her father, Hermann Buck, opposed National Socialism and moved in progressive circles that included Dietrich Bonhoeffer. Buck's mother, Anna Lahusen Buck, was also a woman of conscience. In 1934 Hermann Buck moved his family to a small island in the North Sea, Wangerooge, to escape the disfavor of his Nazi *Gauleiter* or local leader; he had allowed a Black pastor to preach. In Wangerooge Buck would have her first visions.

Those visions took place in 1936, culminating one night on the island's mudflats. She saw two stars rise from the horizon into the night sky, an ascent swifter and brighter than that of any stars she'd ever seen. It was both Holy Thursday and her nineteenth birthday, and Buck passed the night lying in a dune. "I decided," she wrote later, to "allow myself to be led," by the impulses and visions that had recently defined her life.

At dawn, one of the two stars remained in the sky. Buck was moved to walk "precisely on the gleaming trail the star cast upon the wet sand." She came to a tideway near the mudflats, a tideway that always held running water. She fell into it. The bed was muddy, but no water flowed. Workers saw the collapsed teenager and carried her home. She awoke in her own bed.

The experience in the mudflats felt to Buck like a rebirth and on waking, she asked for a piece of cake. Her sister got it for her, but soon Buck's family brought her to a hospital in Jever. She was transferred to Bethel, a Christian psychiatric facility where she would spend the next nine months. Buck was diagnosed with schizophrenia.

In Bethel Buck lived what anyone would define as torture. For as long as twenty-three hours she lay immobilized in "duration baths" that pinned her under tight canvas covers. She was heavily sedated, force-fed, and immobilized at night by icy sheets. The wall of her room held the Gospel words, "Come unto me, all ye who labor and are heavy laden and I will give you rest." Buck called Bethel "a hell amid Bible quotes."

Buck's parents knew Bethel's director, Pastor Friedrich von Bodelschwingh. When Buck was a child, her parents had their children send money to Bodelschwingh as an act of piety, saving by eating rye bread instead of wheat. Buck in childhood helped build the walls of her future prison.

During this stay, Buck was sterilized under the Nazi Hereditary Disease law. For the procedure she was taken from Bethel to a hospital called Gilead; the surgery was passed off as an appendectomy. Buck had dreamt of becoming a kindergarten teacher. Under German law, the sterilized could not attend college or marry the non-sterilized. After her release Buck was despondent, the future she'd imagined lost. She could only, she said later, bear to plan her life one year at a time. She studied pottery, then moved on to clay sculpture. In her art, as in her visions, she allowed herself to feel led. Her recurring subject was the mother and child. In one sculpture, a bending mother's arms spiral into and become the child's. One of her sculptures is still on view in Hamburg, another in Berlin.

Unfortunately, Buck's parents' moral discernment did not reach as far as their daughter's psychiatric treatment. Long after she knew about Buck's abuse at the hands of doctors, her mother wrote her, "you simply must trust the doctor [...]. Just surrender completely to the hands of the experienced doctors and the sooner you will get well again."

Nazi rule had not stopped at sterilization. The hereditary disease law was followed by the 1939 creation of euthanasia programs. These programs aimed to rid the German Reich of the disabled, those they called *Nutzlose Esser*, "useless eaters." The largest of the euthanasia programs, Aktion T4, targeted the neuro-psychiatric. Five gas chambers, the first to be constructed, were built in German asylums. Hitler ended the Berlin-centered T4 program, which kept records and made final death decisions, in August of 1941. Nazis extended the program by decentralizing it and urging personnel at institutions to take the killing into their own hands. This second period was known as "wild euthanasia." Through the euthanasia programs between a quarter million and three hundred thousand died across greater Germany.

Buck learned about the euthanasia murders from the testimony of Nazi Adolf Eichmann when he was captured in 1960 and brought to Israel for trial. Many of the personnel prosecuted for T4 crimes were acquitted; some doctors returned to medical practice. Overwhelmed, Buck put aside her art, writing, "I had the feeling that I alone felt the weight of these dead, these murdered people, because only I cared. [...] I no longer felt motivated to so unconditionally give myself to art."

In March of 1936, before the mudflats, Buck had her first vision. It happened in the family's laundry room. Buck heard three sentences: the first that a war was coming, and it would be "terrible"; the second that she was the Bride of Christ; and the third that one day she would have many things to say and when she did, words would bring themselves forth. Buck turned Cassandra, urging her parents, her choir director, and her doctor to come with her to talk to Hitler, to try to prevent such a terrible war. Her father told her such a war could never happen, her doctor that he could not leave his practice. Her choir director and close friend Molt wrote her that she could accomplish more by focusing on "small things," including her housework.

Buck calls psychosis the result of a "blow to the self," but I include this phrase with the caveat that she would agree all selves experience blows. Her idea of the mind is infinitely creative, and describes a system that heals, with pain and playfulness, from within. In her final psychosis, Buck began to speak what she called an Elementary Language, a linguistic system completely original. The Elementary Language was not static; words changed in response to that which they described. The sounds indicating one tree would reflect the individuality of that tree. When people heard Buck speak this language, they often thought they heard their own tongues: one woman heard Ancient Greek, another Latvian. Buck could speak this language until her death.

In the end, after Buck's fifth psychotic episode in 1959, she had no more. Of this cessation she sometimes uses the language of "healed" or "cured," but here too Buck's definitions are her own. Asked about this language by a correspondent, Buck responded, "For me, my five psychotic episodes were not an 'illness' in the sense of reduction, but the opposite. But because I couldn't achieve my education or my profession in a concentrated way during those times, because my psychosis experiences were more important to me [...] I understand 'healing' in the sense that a person integrates what they experience in psychosis and no longer has to suppress it or split it off."

Buck's life's work was to reimagine the psychotic experience, a reimagining that would lead to a new and holistic doctoring, if it's fair to use that verb, centered around the psychosis-experiencer. In collaboration with psychologist Thomas Bock, she created a system called "trialogue," in which family, clinician, and experiencer meet together as equals. These seminars probed psychosis with the aim of understanding it and limiting, as much as possible, its difficulty. Facilitators and clinicians had to participate as honestly and as vulnerably as all members of the group. Buck was "not a layperson anymore" in her contribution to psychiatry, she writes at the end of *Morning Star;* she experienced her psychosis "too consciously" for that.

Buck explores her trialogue model at the end of *Morning Star.* It began with conversations she'd had with other patients at a dismal psychiatric facility, Ochsenzoll, her last. In the drowsy summer heat, she wrote, eight patients pushed chairs together and discussed their psychoses. They confirmed the value of each other's experiences and the world they shared. They rejected the devaluation they received from their doctors.

Buck encountered Carl Jung's writings after Ochsenzoll, in 1959, and his thinking became important to her. She resonated with Jung's theory that psychosis operates on the level of dream and symbol, including archetypal symbols. Long before any familiarity with Jung, Buck screamed "Unity of Four! Unity of Four!" while being carried down a flight of stairs at Bethel. The quaternity, or unity of four elements, was essential to Jung's concept of a collective symbology. Buck stressed in her writing that psychotics share a visual or imagistic language with one another, a sharing she drew from her fellow patients, her seminars, and her voluminous correspondence. I have experienced this shared imagistic language as well. I did not know German then, when I first encountered Dorothea Buck, but we have always spoken the same language.

It would be a mistake to consider Buck simply a Jungian, or simply someone who leaned psychoanalytic, though she did. For her, psychosis was more than a kind of intense dreaming. The tideway into which she fell had never been free of running water; rather, a few hours before falling, Buck had crossed it by swimming. Visiting Wangerooge, I found a tideway that matched the one she described. It indeed lay too open to the sea to empty all the way to the bottom.

Another Buck hallucination, this one at Bethel, happened in a mind, but also in time and space. The touch of a nurse's hand on Buck's blanket left a spot that spread, turning the blanket red, then fiery hot. Scalding from the blanket left her with boils that had to be healed with x-rays. Patches of Buck's hair fell out. That psychosis existed in its own state of reality was a fact Buck never doubted.

Buck grew up immersed in the world of a pastor's daughter, and Christianity was critical to her thinking. Reconciling the Christian message with what happened to her at Christian institutions like Bethel was a lifelong project. Her spirituality is deeply original. In a letter she describes her activism as a way of giving the divine a means of changing the world. The divine provides to the human "impulses." It is up to us humans who receive these impulses to act in God's place, she wrote, as God is as helpless as a child: "one needs hands and other organs as well as the voice" to act. Buck criticized Christian theologians for accepting artificial social standards of the "norm."

On the Trail of the Morning Star first appeared in 1990. This is the book's first translation into another language. Buck wrote the book as memoir with encouragement from Hans Krieger, a journalist, who later worked with her on the manuscript. Buck had imagined writing a more impersonal work, but Krieger stressed the crucial importance of Buck telling her own story. His importance to Buck is expressed in her acknowledgment.

Buck feared the stigma of others knowing her psychiatric history and published under the alias Sophie Zerchin. Her pseudonym displays typical Buck cheek: it's an anagram for *schizophrenie,* the German word for schizophrenia. Never in any other part of her life—not in her appearances and many protests, her correspondence, her later writings—did Buck use this name. In the second edition of *Morning Star,* she was designated Dorothea Sophie Buck-Zerchin to tie the book and the then-known author together. As Buck did not ever live as Sophie Zerchin, we are acknowledging the woman who lived this life by listing the author's name as Dorothea Buck. We use the pseudonym to remind the reader she was not always able to speak under her own name.

I also want to acknowledge here the generosity of Gabiele Heuer, Fritz Bremer, Hans Krieger, Alexandra Pohlmeier, and Thomas Bock, who gave Buck enormous support when she lived, and helped, in different ways, to shepherd her work and this book into the world. Eva Lipton has been a painstaking and remarkably generous translator.

I published a column recently about the myth that a consciousness like mine, one that leaves consensus reality, can consist only of meaningless brain disease. Almost immediately I received an email from a man who told me I was wrong, that mental illness was a neurological process empty of content, and unattached to the psyche. He let me know he was a mental health expert; I was, as Buck would put it, a layperson. I did not write back, as I have some version of this exchange all the time. Trying to use your voice doesn't override someone else's having removed it. In response to this kind of dialogue, *Morning Star* is a celebratory scream.

Dorothea Buck in 2007 called out psychiatry for following the nosological, category-driven systems set up by Emil Kraepelin. As she pointed out, Kraepelin believed in eugenics and called for "ruthless intervention against hereditary degenerates [...] including use of sterilization." Our current US psychiatry still follows this nosological model, one led by a group of psychiatrists dubbed the "neo-Kraepelinians" by one of their own. This group launched the *Diagnostic and Statistical Manual of Medical Disorders* as we now know it, the book that guides psychiatric diagnosis, practice, and reimbursement.

We still live with a psychiatry marked by symptoms lists, twenty-minute "med checks" with minimal dialogue, and the belief that mental imagery can be purely physiological and meaningless. It is a sad truth that the transformation of psychiatry that Hans Krieger celebrates in his 1990 introduction has never happened. Buck applauded signs of progress throughout her life but always realized far too little has been made. Alternative therapies for the mind—trialogue, medication-free Soteria, the late-eighteenth-century's moral treatment—arise, work well, and never make it to larger practice due to the finances of giving patients more time.

A correspondent wrote Buck in 1994 and asked her about her God figure and her faith. In response she said that she believed "in the certainty that a more insightful and humane psychiatry is not only our concern, but also His. It has to be, or else I would withdraw my allegiance to Him. I envision that we are to be partners with God in making our world more human."

2022

Editor's Foreword to the Paperback Edition

Hans Krieger

Almost nine years have passed since this book was first published. Despite the author's age,[1] she has brought to these years an intense commitment to creating a more humane psychiatry. Not long after the first edition, the author found the courage to remove the pseudonym that had protected her. Under her legal name, Dorothea Buck, Sophie Zerchin has emerged as cofounder of a national self-help association of those involved in the world of psychiatry. She has been a speaker at many conferences. The book has been a guide for many. With the book and with her other actions, Buck has helped see that the new edition comes out amidst better circumstances than the first. Psychiatric progress has come not only from a more refined use of medication and the growth of forms of therapy committed to giving increased attention to the individual. Above all, the willingness to listen to patients, and to take their experiences into account, has grown. Psychosis seminars have increased throughout the country; discussion groups in which professionals, psychiatrists, and family seek a common language

1 Buck was seventy-three when the first edition of *Morning Star* was published. This note and all subsequent notes are by the editor.

and a new understanding of the experience of psychosis. (There is still too little physician participation.) These are encouraging approaches to change, though the medical thinking of medicine still resists it. Today change is also threatened by the lure of genetic research. Dorothea Buck/Sophie Zerchin's book can still do us good service. It still has the character of a groundbreaking venture into territory too little explored.

Munich, 1999

Foreword by the German Publisher

Hans Krieger

We live in an insane world. If the criterion for defining insanity is danger to oneself and one's community, then this declaration needs no further proof. The arsenal of weapons of mass destruction and the alarming progression of the destruction of fundamental necessities of life speak a language all too clear. Yet within this general insanity there is an insanity of a special kind: the so-called madmen, people whose minds seem to function in a way that is beyond the comprehension of "normal" people. They are locked up and undergo treatment against their will until they are inconspicuous enough to fit in. If that is unsuccessful, then they are locked up again.

In early, pre-rational cultures the insane stood close to the divine, their knowledge extending beyond that of the average person. The age of rationality was one of oppression for them; at first the savage oppression of workhouses and idiots' towers,[1] and later the sublime oppression of medicine. The history of psychiatry begins as a history of physical and psychological torture.

Attempts at a more humane treatment developed gradually, constantly threatened by relapses and the danger of slipping into the oppressor's role themselves. This

1 Idiots' towers or fools' towers were common terms for some early European asylums.

cannot come as a surprise, for oppression is inherent in the approach. By being declared ill in a medicinal sense, the insane are deprived of the human significance of their thoughts and feelings. They are viewed and treated like malfunctioning machines. They lose their subject-qualities and become merely objects to be diagnosed, cared for, and stored away.

Seen in this light, the euthanasia murders of the Nazis are, while extreme, a logical consequence of psychiatric ideology. As long as the body's biochemical malfunctions are held responsible for aberrational perception, thinking, and feeling, and the purpose behind such aberrational experiences is not even explored, then any loss of therapeutical optimism must suggest the thought of "life unworthy of life." It is then only the question of moral disinhibition that determines if this thought becomes action. Today the arts of the pharmaceutical industry above all protect us from such consequences, effectively concealing the fundamental failure of classic psychiatry.

Decades of psychiatric research resulted in a plethora of marginal details but no real insight. For example, no one thinking in a purely medicinal sense can say what exactly schizophrenia is, though it is the most commonly diagnosed mental illness.[2] Psychiatrists refuse to decrypt the hidden meaning behind the world-experience of the psychotic. The term itself is misleading. Schizophrenia means "splitting of the mind," yet the schizophrenic person succumbs to their delusions precisely because they cannot achieve the splitting or separation that we do on a daily basis: the separation of the symbolic world of the unconscious from the everyday reality of our rational consciousness. They experience sudden intrusions by subject matter from the unconscious mind, whose symbolic character they misjudge, and must continue to mis-

2 This is no longer true. Depression, anxiety, and other diagnoses are now far more common.

judge as long as their "therapists" do not aid them in the understanding of their symbolic meaning. Attempted suppression of these alien experiences through societal pressure and the chemical bludgeon are far more likely.

Such insight has been made possible by the discovery of psychoanalysis, above all by the school of C.G. Jung. However, headway made in medicine and psychiatric practice through psychoanalytic thinking has been extremely slow, achieving notable standalone results but lacking any widespread effect. Psychiatry, with its custodial practice and purely somatic disease terminology, remained just as resistant here as toward attempts by sociologists and social psychologists to call into question the delimitation between "normal" and "abnormal," therefore relativizing the scale whose gauge defines certain experiences and behaviors as pathological.

Attempts at reform like those of Ronald Laing, Gaetano Benedetti, or Martti Siirala have stimulated theoretical discussion (in Laing's case they even found a lively journalistic echo) but left institutional practices unchanged, at least in Germany. Above all, psychiatry's monopoly on definition remained untouched. Not long ago, learning the nature of their "illness" from the "patients" themselves would have been unthinkable. Standing in the way of this are large-scale reservations, for marginalization and stigmatization of "the insane" also serve the marginalization and suppression of dimensions of experience.

However, recently there have been the first signs of a relaxing of these reservations. Individual psychiatrists, Klaus Dörner for instance, have begun heeding the voices of their patients and wish to learn from them – within certain boundaries, of course. A patients' movement is emerging, not only taking it upon themselves to request from psychiatry a reappraisal of its inhumane past, but also to integrate their own expert knowledge into a psychiatry transformed. For who, if not those affected themselves, can be experts on the question of what "insanity" truly is, how it is experienced, and how one goes about dealing with it?

Sophie Zerchin belongs to the initiators of this patients' movement. Her report gives us an inside look into the psychotic experience. That which seems like pure absurdity from the viewpoint of a psychiatrist, and content-wise would be a waste of time to engage oneself with, reveals itself gradually here as a ciphered pattern of meaningful symbolic coherence that, as soon as it is understood and integrated, does not inhibit life but enriches it. Finding security in a far-reaching, almost cosmic, structure of meaning flashes up again and again in psychotic episodes, as it can never be experienced in the normal state. This truth points out most emphatically that it is not sufficient to see in the psychotic experience simply the effect of a mental defect, of a malfunctioning brain.

At the same time the book documents the inhumanity of psychiatry in its most destructive phase. It documents this rejection of humanity where it hits most directly: in its effect upon the soul of the patient who is already troubled by their initially incomprehensible "delusional experiences" and often deeply disturbed by them. Sophie Zerchin, diagnosed as "schizophrenic," was institutionalized five times. During the Nazi era when she was a young woman, she was forcibly sterilized.

In closing, and this is probably of most importance, Sophie Zerchin escaped from her delusional entanglement under her own power, resulting in an escape from the cycle of institutionalization (an escape from "revolving-door psychiatry," as people like to call it). As she realized that her hallucinations were coming from within herself and desired to be understood symbolically (like the nightly dreams of a "normal" person), she found the key to curing herself. She rejected her medications and became healthy by way of a deepened self-understanding. Her book also gives an account of this, and of the helpfulness of communication with her fellow patients. Contained within is not only a documentation of proving oneself under the most unfavorable conditions, but also the testimony to an extraordinary intellectual achievement.

If an especially gifted person can find and walk the path of healing by achieving understanding through their own intuition, even though everything is designed to ensure their failure, how many others could walk this path if they could find motivated and empathetic support? However, Sophie Zerchin's book is not only a challenge for psychiatry to revise its thinking. It compels us to recognize our idea of "normalcy" as narrow and constrained and invites us to speculate upon a more comprehensive cosmos of human experience.

Sophie Zerchin's self-healing was permanent. A good thirty years have passed since her last psychotic episode, in which the symbolism of her schizophrenia revealed itself to her as a pathway to higher integration. She had understood and did not need another episode. She worked successfully as an artist and teacher and still has the strength in her advanced age for active social commitment, committing herself to the rights of the most disenfranchised in our society: the so-called insane.

Writing a book like this one requires courage. It is still also a risk for someone long healed and well-integrated in society to admit that they were at one time "insane" and an institutional inmate. The power of prejudice is great, and fear of the social consequences of this prejudice is all too justified. Sophie Zerchin's book could and should contribute to the elimination of these barriers.

Munich, March 1990

Introduction by the Author

Sophie Zerchin

Schizophrenia is described in dictionaries as "splitting of the mind." Psychiatric textbooks speak of people who are "disjointed und split." However, in my five psychotic episodes from 1936 to 1959, I never felt split or divided, but rather seized and sometimes overcome by certainties and complexes of meaning, led by an instinct that I experienced as a spontaneous impulse or inner voice. I asked others who, like me, had been diagnosed as "schizophrenic." They too had never felt "disjointed" or "split."

A friend of mine wrote me in 1985:

> Since I was twenty-five years old, I've had diagnosed schizophrenia and have had at least four episodes. During the acute phases of my illness, I never felt split or divided, but rather seized by an unimaginable, fairy-tale apocalyptic complex of meaning that was extremely difficult to live through and consequently pulled me far away from the day-to-day world. The people around me who could only observe my episodes and my confrontations with the demands that were being made of me from the outside must have thought my reactions bizarre or insane. [...] My feeling of life and the world was more like that of a person to whom it suddenly becomes clear that there are deeper floors under their living space and higher ones above

> it; and suddenly these floors that belong to the house that is this person become illuminated from above and below. In this way, the naïve present of life as it was lived suddenly earned a new meaning, in which mythical past rose up to me and religious, apocalyptic visions came crashing down on me. However, this experience contradicts the fundamental experience of disjointedness. If anything, it reflects the experience of a greater unity.

Apparently, many schizophrenics experience these complexes of meaning that they don't feel normally. These can lead to irrational overconfidence and be experienced as paranoia by a person already full of anxiety. For those internally isolated, the experience of a closer connection with the whole can be a great help. Only set against the background of this sensory experience that exceeds the normal state can the ideas of "relationship and meaning" be understood: the symbolic language and actions typical for a schizophrenic. These appear irrational to a psychiatrist because the psychiatrist views them as isolated symptoms and doesn't recognize their hidden contextual meaning.

I wish to help people understand why we who are afflicted cannot disregard our psychotic experience as meaningless and wedge it off from us as something worthless, but rather must come to understand it. Without this understanding, coming from my experience from five episodes, a true and final healing[1] is not possible.

1 A correspondent asked Buck how she used language like "cure" and "healing" given her rejection of the disease model. She replied, "For me, my five psychotic episodes were not an 'illness' in the sense of reduction, but on the contrary. But since I was unable to complete my education or my profession in a concentrated way during those times, because my psychosis experiences were more important to me. [...] I understand 'healing' in the sense that one integrates one's

My first impulse to write was brought about by my horror at the medical murders of over 100,000 institutional patients from 1939 to 1945[2] as well as the inhumane conditions that are still present in our closed institutions. Of my five episodes (1936, 1938, 1943, 1946, and 1959), only the third occurred during the time of "frenzied killings"[3] after the official cessation of patient gassings in August 1941. At that time, I was a patient of the Frankfurt University Neurology Clinic which was under the direction of an opponent of euthanasia, Professor Kleist. Only in passing did I learn of starving patients in the Eichberg asylum in Hesse and could not believe it.

I first heard about the euthanasia victims during the Eichmann trials[4] in 1961. Dismayed, I wanted to learn more. At that time there wasn't anything in the bookstore besides a small chapter in *Doctors of Infamy* by A. Mitscherlich and F. Mielke.[5] I found some important reader's letters in a press archive, among them the letter of a former patient of the Eichberg asylum about his horrific experiences as a pallbearer. The long out-of-print

psychosis experiences and no longer has to split them off from oneself or repress them."

2 Nazi Aktion T4 was a Berlin-centered extermination campaign against the disabled. Among adult victims, the majority were labeled mentally ill. It began in June 1940 and ended in August 1941. After this date the official program ended, but institution directors were encouraged to take the decision to murder into their own hands. Tens of thousands more died. The latter phase is generally called "wild euthanasia."

3 Another term for wild euthanasia.

4 An architect of the Holocaust, Adolf Eichmann was finally captured in Argentina and tried in Israel in 1961.

5 Alexander Mitscherlich and Fred Mielke, eds., *Medizin ohne Menschlichkeit: Dokumente des Nürnberger Ärzteprozesses* (Frankfurt am Main: Fischer, 1960), a paperback reedition of an earlier 1947/1949 publication. The English translation was published as *Doctors of Infamy: The Story of the Nazi Medical Crimes*, trans. Heinz Norden (New York: Henry Schuman, 1949).

account *The Killing of the Mentally Ill in Germany* was lent to me in a roundabout way.[6]

My dismay grew when the *Evangelical Documents on the Murder of the "Incurably Ill" under the National Socialist Regime from the Years 1939–1945* appeared.[7] Since the end of the 1950s, I had been working as a sculptor on public commissions which could only be won through competitions and would have needed my undivided attention for my work. Yet the suppressed patient murders and the inhumanity of our institutions troubled me so deeply that I found myself pulled away from my artistic work to the typewriter again and again. The focus of my artistic work was the relationship between shapes and forms; the lack of relation these psychiatrists felt toward their patients went against all semblance of humanity, without which I feel there could be no art. I was unable to force myself to the other side of this abyss of indifference, and I didn't want to, either. Only we who have lived this would be able to contribute more insight and humanity to psychiatry – and only by refusing to remain mute victims and objects.

Because of the acquittals of many thousands of medical murderers owing to "unlawfulness unable to be proven without a doubt" – reported in Frankfurt in 1967 to "frenetic applause from the audience" – we who were targeted came to realize that the murders committed on institutional patients did not count as crimes in our "constitutional state." The doctors who took part in the murders from institutions, health departments, and universities remained well regarded. We, on the other hand, remained the "inferiors." Each person remained alone

6 Alice Platen-Hallermund, *Die Tötung Geisteskranker in Deutschland* (Frankfurt am Main: Verlag der Frankfurter Hefte, 1948). This book was reprinted in 1993 by Psychiatrie-Verlag in Bonn.

7 Evangelische Kirche in Deutschland, *Evangelische Dokumente zur Ermordung der „unheilbar Kranken" unter der nationalsozialistischen Herrschaft in den Jahren 1939–1945*, ed. Hans Christoph von Hase (Stuttgart: Evangelisches Verlagswerk, 1964).

with their knowledge of these crimes. I was first able to free myself from the burden of this knowledge and from my rage at our powerlessness by writing a play called *The Tragedy of Euthanasia.*[8]

The commitment of some journalists since the 1960s who consistently confront the public with our misery in the institutions, especially in the publications *Stern, Spiegel,* and *Zeit,* was encouraging. I would especially like to remember Frank Fischer, who got himself hired in various institutions and first reported his to some extent appalling experiences in *Zeit* and then in his 1969 book *Insane Asylums: Patients Accuse.*[9]

In the twenty years that have passed since then there have been some reforms. Nevertheless, Uwe Heitkamp and Michael Herl,[10] who allowed themselves to be committed to various institutions in multiple states, give an account in ARD Report:

> It seems to me that there is hardly a hope for them on the inside, and that has been for years and decades. They are observed, monitored, locked up, and pumped full of medications. The continuous dimmed lighting day and night causes headaches. The bed equipment is perfect: hand bindings, ankle cuffs, and waist straps are mounted within easy reach on the bed.

An employee of *Zeit,* Hans Krieger, had advocated a more understanding treatment of psychotic patients in dedi-

8 This play is a collage of material related to the medical trials. It includes real people involved with the trials and the crimes. Buck laments that no one is interested in the murder of the "sick." The fact that the play was never performed unfortunately proved her right.

9 Frank Fischer, *Irrenhäuser: Kranke klagen an* (Munich: Kurt Desch, 1969).

10 Uwe Heitkamp and Michael Hert are German investigators and documentarians.

cated reviews of psychiatric and psychological literature. He introduced us to psychiatrists like Jan Foudraine and Ronald Laing who were trying to understand schizophrenia from the patient's perspective. I got in touch with Hans Krieger through my younger sister. I followed up the *Euthanasia* play with a manuscript in which I dealt with the somatic dogma of the psychiatric doctrine and pled for a psychological understanding of the psychotic experience.

After reading the first part of my manuscript, Hans Krieger wrote me:

> Nowadays there is a lot of literature criticizing psychiatry that has brought up many intelligent and important points. But there are always psychiatrists and other laymen out there expressing their opinions. The experts (I mean the patients, the people who have experienced psychosis themselves) are never asked and are seldom able to have a voice. They, as people with their own experiences, are far more important than any theory. It doesn't happen often that a person is able to free themselves from psychosis while also understanding what happened during it; and the fact that you also have the gift of writing is serendipitous. I would think it a waste if you contented yourself with writing something that a psychiatrist or a journalist also could.

But could I give an account of my psychosis so openly and unreservedly as he had proposed? Would I not come to regret having divulged such intimate things? Every derogatory judgment concerning the "insane" troubles me deeply still to this day. Apart from that, the murders of those who suffered with me and the injustice of my forced sterilization weighed heavy on me. If the dogmatic prejudice of psychiatrists could lead to such crimes, then something had to finally happen to open their eyes. And they could only come to know the reality of what we underwent through our own experiences.

For a year and a half, I let the matter rest. Then I concluded that I should write down my experiences as an institutionalized patient. I hope my account contributes to the better understanding and more respectful treatment of those undergoing psychosis.

Hamburg, 1990

1

Rebirth on the Mudflats

On April 9, 1936, I felt myself driven out into the dunes. It was Holy Thursday — I was born on a Holy Thursday nineteen years before. It was late afternoon when I left home. For some weeks, I had been experiencing these strong inner impulses. I followed them without question, for to me they felt like the guidance of the words of Paul: "Those who are guided by the spirit of God are the sons of God."[1]

I spent the night in the hollow of a dune. It was cold. From time to time, I climbed up the dune to watch the first and then the second star appear over the horizon of the mudflats. Was it Venus and Mercury? It was a wonder to me that a star could ascend from the horizon high up into the sky in a single night, as the morning star does here. I had never seen it happen, never heard or read about it. Perhaps it is rare to see it in this position and so be able to follow its full course.

At dawn, as the star stood high in the sky, I took off my things, my favorite sweater and everything else, and buried them in the sand. The end of my vanity. All that I kept on was my winter coat. Then I went after the morning star that John had identified at the end of his revelations with Jesus. At first, I walked along the embankment, then

1 Romans 8:14.

onto the mudflats. I walked precisely on the gleaming trail the star cast upon the wet sand. I had been waiting to set out and now understood the meaning behind this foreshadowing sign of a development with which I had to catch up.

I came to a tideway that never dried up, even when the tide was at its lowest. I knew about it from a mudflat hike in the summer. We had had to cross it, and despite the low tide the water had come up to our hips both times. Now I had to swim through the tideway. The morning star faded as I reached the other shore. Only the moon, which stood next to it, was still visible. I had stumbled into a spot with deep mud. I took off my coat and kicked it under my feet, but I still sank deep into the mud. And then the moon faded too. What should I do now? *Help me please, Jesus, I'm freezing,* I begged, exhausted from the cold, sleepless night.

I turned myself around toward the island and fixed my gaze on the lighthouse. But there, where just before I had had to swim, the water was now gone. I crawled on all fours back through the mud, pulled myself up onto a big, egg-shaped buoy, looked behind myself once more, saw the sun rise, and lost consciousness.

I was lying at home in the light of my mother's presence. Workers had found me. I could no longer understand any of it; the miracle of the star was just as beyond my comprehension as the dry tideway bed. At first, I asked myself if they were all angels. Were miracles still occurring every day, and had I been the only one not to know about it? When I told my mother that I had seen a star ascend from the lowest point on the horizon high up into the sky and after that a second one, she shook her head in disbelief: that could not be. Because of that, I decided not to tell her about the second miracle, that the tideway bed had been without water.

Despite that, I wanted to celebrate this day festively—with a piece of cake. My sister fetched it from the baker immediately. I was convinced that this was the most important day of my life: the day of my rebirth from the tidal mud. I still wore this mud as a dried-up black crust on my skin, and as it was being scrubbed off in the bath, my knee emerged, cut up by seashells. That was the proof that I had crawled back and not swum, I thought. And it could also have proven the miracle in the spot where my coat had sunk: exactly where the lines between lighthouse and buoy intersected with the far bank of the tideway shore. That's where I would find it. I must have been discovered at the big buoy that lies on the island side of the tideway, covered in a layer of mud that would have been washed away while swimming. Like a real birth, I thought: instead of the waters of birth being washed away, it's the water of the tideway.

Some weeks before, I had been walking beside the sea. The sand was hard, and the going was easy. Above the bright gray water with its dark, outreaching breakwaters, the indistinct light of the sun floated behind the fog — a weightless, almost serene sight. I didn't want to walk the same way twice and I climbed up the chain of dunes to walk back along the mudflats. Sea and mudflats live off the sky that they reflect, and, depending upon the color of the clouds, it is often a stunning image. This time the image was one of disconcerting gloom.

Like a long-dead force, the mudflats lay unmoving in the gray fog, in odd contrast with the sea under the floating light of the overcast sun. With every step I sank into the soft, wet, grass-covered ground. A seagull lifted off from the ground and sank immediately back down. Another lay dead by a tide pool between the rushes. The path stretched endlessly alongside the ruler-straight embankment.

The next morning this path had turned into music for me. Music began with the foghorn. Polyphony entered with the sun's theme, floating unseen behind the fog. The dark breakwaters, reaching far out into the sea, sounded up from the depths, as if to hold the floating light. I could hardly keep up notating the music as I heard it well up inside me. I of course had no fitting notes for the music, so I simply traced the melodic arcs with my pencil. I wanted to be able to draw them clearly later and assign each voice a different color.

Then came the climb up the chain of dunes. The looming dark power of death weighed heavily upon the mudflats. And exactly this section of the music inspired me: the collision of two opposing powers as the climax. Yet right here at the most thrilling section, from one beat to the next, the music suddenly stopped. Nothing more could be heard, not a single sound. I despaired.

Had it been a secret fear that caused the music to break off abruptly at its climax? The fear that my life's path would end up following prescribed, tired routines, just like the path running along the ruler-straight embankment? And had that same fear forced me to follow the bright trail that the morning star cast in the wet sand during the dawn of Good Friday? Exactly at the same spot, just like the first time, the seagull had flown up from the tide pool beside the embankment and descended again, as if an oppressive weight lay upon it. But this time I had seen the radiant sun rising above the mudflats, and the sun transformed everything. My experiencing of the world in symbols, which would come to dominate my psychotic phases, began with this "life's path" transformed into music.

This event was fundamental for me and wasn't "insane" in my eyes at all. Biblical accounts like Abraham's Test of Faith showed clearly enough that divine guidance was something completely different from our everyday reason. Wasn't the unwavering faith in God supposed to have the power to move mountains? If God had required Abraham to sacrifice his dearest and only child, why shouldn't He have required me to overcome myself, as the thing dearest to me?

That was the intrusion of the otherwise unconscious into the conscious—an intrusion of another reality, the symbolic reality. Psychiatry views such an intrusion as an illness, an illness called "schizophrenia." That term describes a division, a division between dreamworld and external reality. However, I never felt divided in my psychotic episodes, but, rather, had a deeper feeling of coherency.

In a "normal" state, I never would have felt myself driven to follow the trail of the morning star in the wet mud. But then I would also never have experienced my symbolic birth. I wasn't aware of the fact that I would experience it when I set off into the mudflats.

An Easter rabbit picture book arrived for me with the Easter Sunday post, without a return address. I was delighted that someone had thought to give it to me for my rebirth and I looked through it attentively. Then I was laid on a woven stretcher with a cover, like one might use to transport sick people by ship. Rebirth is followed by the baby basket, I thought.

In a barred room at the mainland hospital, I was disabused of associations of this nature. Here, where I was supposed to stay for the Easter holidays, it was eerie. For me, the eeriness was embodied by the fact that no one spoke to me. I had come along trustingly, and now I had been put behind bars, and no one told me why. The lawbreaker understands the reasons behind their imprisonment, but the so-called insane person doesn't know why they're being locked up.

The hospital seemed to be barely occupied over the Easter holidays. A nurse came in, but she didn't speak to me. At night she kept watch in the adjoining room. The little window between us through which she could watch me remained illuminated all through the night. Easter Sunday was a dreary, rainy day. A heavy silence stretched out, punctuated every quarter hour by the ringing of a bell from the nearby castle tower. A colorful goldfinch sat upon the balcony parapet in front of the window. Could it be the one that flew away from me years ago? Grown so round in the time that had passed? Orderlies and nurses made a game of teasing me, so I grabbed the necklace of one of the nurses, possibly ripping it.

What was I doing here? I had spent the previous night following the star's ascent. My mother had declared that impossible, but what was impossible was that I could have been wrong. Had the Miracle of Christmas Night happened again, and I was the only one to see it? No, that could not be; the observatories were still there. Now I was being punished for witnessing a miracle on the mudflats. I just couldn't comprehend it. And so my fear grew and grew in this eerie silence that surrounded me.

Why had no one from home come with me? Why had they let me be taken to this dismal hospital and left me without any further consideration? And what was the purpose of this card they had given me with the Bible verse, "Yea, though I walk through the valley of the shadow of death, I will fear no evil."[2] I had walked through no such dark valley. I had experienced a miracle: my own rebirth. They had only brought me into a dark valley by sticking me in this hospital and leaving me all alone. And they hadn't even told me where I was going.

Anger was now added to fear. I ripped up the card with the verse as well as the Easter rabbit book. I threw the Easter eggs and the oranges that they had given me at the room's walls. Then I tipped the large iron grate, which was only tied up at the top, out of the window frame, blocking the door. I shoved my bed in front of it. The orderlies should at the least have to stay outside my room. I probably also ripped the curtains. But the orderlies came, nevertheless. One stood on the balcony in front of the door; the other two in front of the grate at the door.

2 Psalm 23:4.

I swung my bedpan threateningly, but they forced their way into my room holding a syringe. I struck one of them in the head with the bedpan, and of course it hit the one who had been friendly and never teased me. They shoved the anesthetic syringe into my thigh and then forced me down into the cellar.

"Unity of Four! Unity of Four!" I screamed on my way down the stairs. That was my protest against being punished for the miracle on the mudflats by being locked up, sedated, and detained in the basement. It was simultaneously my protest against a trinity that we the afflicted are excluded from, because the Spirit of God cannot work within us.

The "Unity of Four" remained a central theme of my psychosis: the union of Spirit and Nature, God and World. It gained great meaning especially during my fifth episode in 1959. I later found an explanation in C.G. Jung's work. What I called "Unity of Four," he called *quaternity*. Quaternity is one of the great symbols of unity. Jung writes:

> When the fourth variable joins the other three, the "One" emerges, which symbolizes complete unity. In analytic psychology, it is frequently the lower functions (i.e., the functions that the conscious mind cannot control) that the "Fourth" embodies. Its integration into consciousness is the main task of the process of individuation.[3]

The basement was pitch black. They had laid me on a mattress on the ground. I crawled along the wall in the darkness until I felt two small mortarboards. I laid them on my body crosswise and felt calmer, drifting into sleep. The orderly whom I had struck in the head with the bed-

3 Aniela Jaffé, ed., *Erinnerungen, Träume, Gedanken von C.G. Jung* (Zurich and Düsseldorf: Walter Verlag, 1993), 414.

pan came by in the morning. “Take a look, that’s the spot where you hit me!” He showed me a large purple bruise on his forehead. I truly was sorry. I hadn’t wanted to hit him.

The father of my friend Armgard came by later, as well as the district nurse who had accompanied me on the ship. They pulled a pair of woolen knickers over my nightgown, tucked me into my old winter coat, and tied my hands together. So now I was dangerous, apparently. I sat with the district nurse in the back seat of the car. Armgard’s brother, who was being driven by his father to the Deacon’s School, sat up front. During the drive I tried to loosen the ties around my wrists a little bit to shove my hat back into place, since it had slid down onto my face. That was reason enough to give me another injection. It felt like a punishment. Once again, I had no idea where I was being brought.

2

Childhood and Crisis

How does schizophrenia develop? Does it spring up from the course of life, from ways of reacting that were already developed during childhood? Perhaps to compensate for the feeling that something is missing? With the way my childhood played out, I could imagine that.

I was born during World War I. My father "stood in the field," as they said back then. What kind of field could that have been that my father was standing in? His cot stood folded up in the attic—it was our emergency bed, taken along with every move. I had it later in my first small studio, the only piece of furniture there besides my modeling stand and a borrowed stool for my portrait models.

Father needed the cot, since he worked as a traveling priest[1] with no permanent shelter. There's a yellowing photo with me sitting on his lap. It's my first birthday. The garden arbor we're sitting in is still bare, but I have a wreath of primroses on my head. My father looks happy and is smiling. I am too. In later pictures of me I always look somewhat sad. He is holding me gently, but one can

1 Buck's father Hermann Buck was a Protestant pastor. He was staunchly anti-Nazi. Hermann Buck relocated from Saxony after falling afoul of the local Nazi *Gauleiter* for allowing a Black pastor to preach. The family relocated to the island of Wangerooge, in the North Sea, where Buck experienced rebirth on the mudflats.

see that it's been a long time since I've been in his arms. He's wearing a simple soldier's uniform. My parents had actually hoped to have a boy, so that my brother, two years older, could have a playmate. Since they already had two girls.

We were never playmates, my brother and me. I had hardly begun to tell a story: "Once upon a time there was a bunny...," when he immediately cut me off: "...who had a little snub nose." He meant me; I was the one with the little snub nose. But I didn't want to tell a story about me, but rather about the bunny, who would play such a large role in my fictitious childhood.

On this first birthday it may have only been the second time my father had ever seen me. When the war ended and he came home again, I was one and a half. That's what he blamed the gulf that lay between us on. He devoted the entirety of his love to my younger sister who was born three years after me. There wasn't enough left over for me, I felt, and therein lay the grief that overshadowed my entire childhood and accompanied me far beyond it.

My mother tried to balance out this lack of love for me but that seemed to aggravate my three older siblings. They allowed father's special love for our youngest; they even seemed to share in that feeling. However, they couldn't tolerate my mother favoring me. The age gap between us was probably not big enough for that either.

One time I dreamed mother had drowned. I awoke in the dark and knocked on my parents' door. I had to make sure right away that mother was still there. She opened the door in her nightgown, but then I didn't dare tell her that I had dreamed something so terrible about her. She was somewhat annoyed that I had woken her in the middle of the night for no reason. Maybe she drowned in my dream because my father always called her *Entchen*, "duckling." I didn't realize he was actually saying *Ännchen*, "Annie," until later.

Being loved less than my younger sister weighed heavily on me. Still heavier was the conclusion that I was less worthy of love. I myself thought I was "catty," as they said back then, but I noticed early on this had something to do with my unhappy position within our family. As a small child I had been considered especially cheerful. I sought a substitute in intensive play, and somehow, even while playing, I felt that I continued to flee from something.

In the 1920s playing could still truly be one's purpose in life, since automobiles hadn't yet forced us children off the streets and schools left sufficient time for play. Many games had their dedicated season. During the time of the spinning top game, children could be seen everywhere on flat, paved surfaces pulling along their colorful wooden spinning tops with a string on a stick. During the marble game season, they could be seen throwing colored clay marbles or the larger ones made of lead or glass into troughs on unpaved roadsides. Swap jumping, peg book, and the hopscotch game "Hinkepinke" also had their own seasons. Only girls played these three games, while knifing was a common game among boys. An open pocketknife would be thrown into a box sketched in the soil, and the blade sticking in the ground would show which direction the box would be divided in until one player was king of the entire box. The games unbound to the seasons were played in our garden, the meeting spot for many of the children from our street. Farmers still lived all around the city.

When I think back, I have the feeling that my parents also found playing more important than school. Since I was considered delicate, being a child born during the war, they often let me skip school. My mother homeschooled me during my first school year, despite having almost no time with a large household and five children. But I would have much rather attended school. The schoolyard bordered on our land behind the garden, and a beekeeper had his hives in a wooden frame there. Every day I would sit there on a covered board with a sandwich and a cup of warm milk for my brother who would come up to the fence during recess. In the end it was agreed that each time a female student was absent I would be allowed to take her place. One day I came home disappointed: everyone had been present again. But there was one girl with a swollen cheek; she would definitely be absent tomorrow.

When I started attending school regularly in my second year, however, its initial charm had somewhat lessened for me. I barely remember anything from all my elementary school years, except drawing little Easter eggs in a new notebook and coloring them in, instead of having to draw them on the chalkboard. And the teacher (she was a cousin of my father) with her red-blonde hair and bright blue eyes; she was strict, but when she spoke her mouth looked kind. I have a precise memory only of things that left a great impression upon me. That's why I have such a good memory for the unusual things I experienced in my psychotic phases while forgetting much of what transpired in the time in between. My experiences during psychosis left a fundamental impression.

Mother had run a daycare center with a friend before her marriage. Because of that, she had a well-developed sense of how much time children needed for play. Father shared her view, so we grew up practically without worrying about school. We also barely needed to help out around the house. Around noon we would dry off twenty or thirty dishes (the number would be negotiated when we ate); Saturdays we would rake the garden pathways (which we felt was a lot of work); and get bread and milk if the milkman's horse cart hadn't brought enough. There were probably only a few parents at that time who believed playtime played such a large role in childhood development.

Father, being so open-minded in one area, showed far less psychological understanding in others, and I grappled with that. He ascribed certain traits to us children, put a stamp on us. Because of this, a hierarchy developed among us — one that could also become a pecking order. "My oldest sister is smart, the second one is beautiful, and I have nothing," I said gloomily to an aunt of mine (she told me about it later). I didn't come away completely empty-handed, though. Father thought I was "guileless" and that I wrote and spoke "openly about whatever comes into my head." He even thought I would "be the first to marry."

But that was only a small consolation for me. I didn't feel like it was true appreciation, because he gave that to my three smarter sisters. My lack of logic made him impatient. In the end, I would barely even dare open my mouth at the dinner table in case I said something illogical. For that reason, I had to learn Latin, because it apparently helps teach logical thinking. I even had fun learning it, but I don't think it made me more logical. Today it actually astounds me that I was considered the most ungifted in the family, because at the end of my schooling I was among the seven best students out of forty, despite the amount of time I missed.

I was also not a great beauty. My father would sometimes call my broad nose a "witch's dance floor." He meant it as a joke, but it didn't feel that way to me at all. I comforted myself with that fact that he would sometimes call me "Egyptian Princess" — also because of my nose. He had lived in Jerusalem and Alexandria for a long time. That's where he and mother had met. I sought to balance the scales with my younger sister. If father and my older siblings loved her so much more than me, then she should at least love me the most. I pestered her over and over, asking whom she loved most after our parents.

I especially loved my dolls. When we were out of town, I wrote them loving letters. Even as a twelve-year-old I wished for a doll, and she became my favorite. She had to learn Latin, just like me. From time to time, however, I would switch her personality back and forth between schoolgirl and baby. My older siblings disapproved; they thought the steady development from three-year-old to schoolboy that my younger sister gave her boy doll was far more proper. But I needed those baby phases. The memory of the wicker doll carriage lined with flowered fabric where my doll would rest swaddled, and the warm children's room with the large-tiled stove and snow-covered garden outside the windows — even today this makes me feel a childlike comfort that I'm hard-pressed to find anywhere else in my memory.

In the summer, our dolls lived in a garden house that father carpentered. The garden, with its long hedge and many bushes, offered so many hidden nooks and crannies; the large, mysterious cellar; and the double attic with its rubbish-filled corners that ignited my imagination — these made up the kingdom my younger sister and I played in. In the coal cellar we and our girlfriends built a mountain of briquettes that we hid in. In the large, white-tiled kitchen, which was only used for canning, we picked out what we needed for our games from among discarded household appliances. In the adjacent canning cellar, there was once a large carboy with apple juice. Each of us had hidden a jar there, and our unsuspecting mother marveled at how quickly the carboy became empty. The elevator that led from the canning cellar to the dining room above on a thick rope thrilled us: again and again we would heave ourselves up and come flying back down, until the game was decided to be too dangerous, and we had to stop. A popular hiding place was the apple cellar with its stored winter fruit on long shelves. The laundry room, with its walled-in wash kettle and wooden tub attracted me because of its strange smell. The old chicken coop, on the other hand, I avoided, because even though we no longer kept them, I thought it still smelled like chickens. I often dreamed that a hunchbacked little man lived in it. There was also an old iron tripod over which father had soled our shoes.

The most mysterious room was the dim potato cellar. Through a tarnished little window thin light fell from a room in front of it that was only accessible from outside. What might be hidden there was an unsolvable riddle that stoked the most adventurous ideas. But one day the room was open from the outside door and the magic was gone: there were just old boxes in it.

The double attic, however, kept its magic. The suspended floor above the spacious drying loft could only be climbed using a huge bed crate. From there we could climb through a roof hatch onto a small platform on the roof. Then we would settle in with some pillows and enjoy the view. One day, however, we saw the bearded elder of the church office running toward the house, quite out of breath. I had never seen this otherwise bulky man so agitated. He came to tell my father that we were on the roof, and from then on, we were forbidden from going up there.

My mother, on the other hand, calmly accepted my clothes constantly being ripped from climbing trees. As I began climbing during a family outing, I slipped from the tree and scraped up my legs. That hurt a lot, but then I lay for some days in the room directly beside my father's workroom. I had never seen him so concerned about me. No wonder I wanted to fall from more trees after that. It didn't happen.

In the garden and cellar I never felt at a disadvantage — they were our kingdom. In contrast, my memory avoids our actual living spaces, except for during holidays. Nowhere were Advent, Christmas, Easter, and Pentecost, but also Sunday morning — there was homemade white bread and apple jelly — celebrated as festively as with us. What is now called an "idyllic world" took place in these rooms. Every Sunday, and as often as my father found time during the week, our family gathered around the large round mahogany table in the living room after dinner to play games or read aloud. Fritz Reuter was my father's favorite to read aloud. Fontane, Wilhelm Raabe, and Gustav Freytag's *Soll und Haben* were of course also part of the family reading list. That I didn't want to read all these books was something father disapproved of. I could only imagine them being boring. *Soll und Haben*—that sounded far too stuffy.

It delighted me when father sometimes played at being a sheep for us at table. He would brush his thin, fine hair into his face, looking adorably stupid with his wide-open, astonished eyes and half-opened mouth. I wish he could have always been so funny and easygoing. He was forty-five years older than me and usually just an authority figure.

My adventurousness often broke the boundaries of what was allowed. My friend from elementary school and I loved adventurous explorations, which my parents found too dangerous and forbade. Once, when my parents were out of town, we went on a pilgrimage to an old robbers' den far outside the city that our teacher had told us about in local history class. We were disappointed to find no robbers there, just playing children. Some years later, instead of robbers, we sought the heroes of prohibited mystery novels. We hid them in our schoolbooks and devoured them secretly.

When we were twelve and first allowed to attend the opera, it was Weber's[2] *Der Freischütz* (*The Marksman*), we were especially impressed by wicked Kaspar. For days my high school friend and I walked up and down below the singer's windows. Finally, the sleeveless arm of a man reached out and pulled a towel inside that had been drying on the window handle. His arm! We were satisfied but also a bit disillusioned, and we stopped our daily walks. Listening raptly to his vocal exercises and arias had lost its charm for us. The rest of the class stuck with good Max.

2 Carl Maria von Weber was a German composer.

The older brother of this friend was also my first love, even though he of course didn't pay any attention to a twelve-year-old. I admired his helpfulness: at home he hauled coal for their stove. When I got tired on a long school sledding trip on the frozen meadows, he pushed me back across ditches that crackled alarmingly in the darkness. I was enraptured when my friend showed me a photo of him: he was wearing a white robe and a laurel wreath in his dark curls—his class was performing a Greek play. One time, as I was heading to my relatives and the train was going past his house, I suddenly got a fierce stomachache. So this was how unrequited love made itself known!

Every morning when I woke up, I would immediately think of something to look forward to. When I was fourteen, however, this method had stopped working. The game had lost its charm and nothing new had come to take its place. A vague sadness overcame me. I talked to my mother about it.

"Don't take yourself so seriously," was her response. But how was doing nothing supposed to help me? Being able to do something had always been what I loved about life. Since I had been young, I had always hurled myself into activities in order to forget and suppress my feelings of disadvantage. If I did or planned nothing, sadness would overcome me. In a hidden corner of the garden, I would breathe my sadness into my harmonica, and yet at the same time I would have preferred to just come out and say what I was feeling.

Back then, we children each had our own garden with a young apple or pear tree, with flowers, radishes, and cress that we tended ourselves. My three older siblings had a larger one, we "two little ones" a more modest one. And in each garden stood an arbor made of wire mesh, entwined with vetches or nasturtiums. Once we were sitting with our parents, spread out among the five arbors having lunch, when it suddenly occurred to me that there was something important I didn't know yet. "Mother, where do little children actually come from?" I called over to her. She was sitting in another arbor, but I naturally expected her to call back the answer just as spontaneously and nonchalantly as me. The thought that my question was embarrassing or inappropriate then and there didn't even occur to me.

Now I was fourteen, and I began to see the world through different eyes. Many things now moved me that I had hardly noticed before. In the early morning darkness on the way to school, I was enchanted by a young tree with countless raindrops shimmering on its branches in the whitish light of a streetlamp. Adalbert Stifter's *Nachsommer* and the Worpswede painters Paula Modersohn-Becker and Heinrich Vogeler began to replace the opera singer I had idealized before. But simply empathizing and admiring wasn't enough for me. I had to do something; I needed a replacement for our games.

By the time I was twelve, I knew I wanted to be a kindergarten teacher, and so I came up with the idea for a games and crafts circle for children. This was a pretty audacious idea since I was still just a child myself, but my parents agreed to the plan, so I asked some families from an apartment complex if their children would want to come on Sunday afternoons to play and do crafts. In the beginning, thirteen children came, later the circle grew to twenty-eight between the ages of four and fourteen. Before Christmas, even some of the parents came to help with making toys.

A friend, whom I'm still friends with today, helped me with this improvised kindergarten. On an outing where we had taken our old pot-bellied baby carriage for the littlest kids to ride in, after delivering the group back to their homes, my friend spontaneously climbed into the high-wheeled carriage, covered with flowering jasmine branches, and I rushed off, pushing her through town.

This massive baby carriage, the likes of which I've never seen since, was stowed away in a chicken wire cage to protect it from cats and other animals. It was definitely characteristic of my parents' vision for raising children: even when we were babies, we were supposed to have as much room to roam as possible while still being carefully shielded from any conceivable danger.

But for me there remained a recurring reactionary behavior: the desire to make up for a feeling of lacking something through activity. First the intense playing, later the children's playgroup — both these were intended to help me overcome this painful feeling of disadvantage.

In the meantime, we had moved to an island. I loved the freedom of our lifestyle there. Prior to this, my self-confidence had been strengthened during a year in a women's boarding school, where I had been fully acknowledged. The relationship to my father had also gotten closer due to the weekly correspondence with my parents. The sense of discrimination was something I shouldn't have had to deal with at this point, for my father wrote to me: "My dearest mouse, someone who can write letters like yours is certainly not boring! They are interesting and funny and smart and so much more!" To be considered intelligent by Father must have made me feel very good.

It was a happy year in the new home. Just my younger sister and I, as well as a "house daughter" finishing high school and who became a friend, were left at home. We ran the house for a year. Once we finished the lunch dishes, the afternoon belonged to us. Following the wind, we ran along the wide beach, which was empty once the summer months were over. In order to zip alongside the water even faster I thought up something: I removed the wheels from my old doll carriage and strapped them to my feet and then used a sail to let the wind push me. But the wheels should have had ball bearings and wider rubber wheels. I drew a design for roller skates with windsail power: under each foot two wheels between metal tracks on which the shoe could be strapped. I sent the drawing to a company and was very proud with the answer, which began with the salutation, "Dear Mr. ...." I took that as recognition — apparently one did not assume a girl could have such an idea.

That was in 1935. I met Molt in the fall of this year and that must have been the start of the conflict which would trigger my psychosis. Together with my mother, my girlfriend Armgard, and her parents, I had a singing retreat on the island. Molt was the choral director: I can still see myself walking toward the participants with Armgard. They descended from the boat in a long row and walked between the rails of the little island railway: deacons, unaffiliated nuns, community helpers, also two ministers, and a vicar, so there was a total of twenty-five of us. Loaded down with baggage they balanced from one railway tie to the next while we let our bare feet touch the shallow water unencumbered.

Molt, like his wife, dragged a heavy suitcase, dressed in a gray trench coat and a beret. Suddenly I felt his gaze on me. This unsettled me. I did not know what to think of him. I did not think he was nice but at the same time he impressed me. Over the course of the retreat my initial dislike disappeared. While conducting, he at times seemed to turn inward in a way I had not seen before. His movements were contained but he exuded great inner vitality and a sense that he had a great range of human possibility. At the same time, he seemed unconventional, which I especially noticed in this circle of people. He apparently put a lot of importance on celibacy, which he referred to constantly when teaching us an old folksong he particularly liked.

We were fulfilled by the communal singing and living. But on the second to last day — the entire retreat community was at our house — Molt became "blood brothers" with our dachshund. He did this with a piece of sugar, and it was done in jest. However, I could not see the fun in it. To be brothers with a dog—I could somehow imagine that. But blood brothers? Didn't Molt devalue his own human nature with that? From the start I had been unsettled that he showed his feelings, but also seemed to feel guilt at feeling the way he did. Or was it exactly this paradox that was the source of his vitality?

Molt was supposed to return the end of January 1936, this time just for the islanders. Knowing this made me happy. The end of January—it was only a few months until then. I advertised this second singing retreat enthusiastically to our friends. The young middle school teacher looked at me with amusement as I rhapsodized about Molt and singing together.

Happily, Armgard and I picked Molt up from the island train station. He would stay for four days; in the mornings, Armgard and I were supposed to each have a half-hour individual lesson with him. In the afternoons and evenings, the whole choir would sing.

"You are shining like the sun," Father commented during mealtime. I was sitting next to Molt. I had felt timid with him during the first choral retreat and had silently changed my seat when I saw the name card with his name next to my seat. I handed him a dish. His hand recoiled. "I can't touch things that are so hot," he said. "We can, we are reformed," I responded jokingly. "A big word," he guessed. "You aren't smart?" he asked me during a singing lesson. "No." I could admit it without a second thought, because he was the kind of person with whom being smart had not developed its own dynamic: thinking, feeling, and imagination seemed to be balanced in him, I thought. This first interaction with a true artist had something liberating for me. And his interest in me also felt good.

The penultimate evening following the choir singing, we went to the beach: Molt, Armgard, and I. The ocean was alight with fireflies. A glowing ocean on a January night! I only knew summer evenings to be like this. Above us the starry sky and next to us the shimmering ocean. We were elated and happy and very young. I was eighteen, Armgard two years older, Molt thirty-three. "Girls, take me in between you!" he said. Arm-in-arm we walked along the oceanside and he spoke to us of the breadth of Christianity, which was so much broader than the narrow pastor-focused church. I was very impressed by how alive Jesus was for him.

The next morning, however, it was as if the ground had been pulled from under my feet. The most important thing I felt was missing. "I can't sing anymore," I said during the singing lesson, "everything is broken." "And it's my fault!" he said. "Fault?" I asked. "You are now the fourth for whom I've destroyed everything," he responded. "And then I will leave again and leave you alone. I don't know whether I am allowed to do that."

"You must do it," I said. For I hardly thought it was in his power to stop since it wasn't his words which had moved me but the whole person. "What happened to the others?" I wanted to know. They had all been older than me, already had careers. A district nurse lived with him and his wife for half a year and was deeply moved by the inner breadth of their Christianity.

"Why is it you are so sad / and don't even laugh. / I see it in your eyes / that you've cried..." In the end I did learn this song.

The last song evening was over. We'd sat together. "Now we are gods and will ascend Olympus," Molt said as we mounted the steep stairway, and he took me in his arms encouragingly. I felt everything other than Olympian. The next morning his ship would be leaving.

"What are you doing?" he asked the next morning as I was sweeping the hallway. I took this last opportunity for a conversation. "What does it mean to be a Christian?" I asked. "To take God's hand," he answered. I thought I had taken his hand since the first days of my childhood. I loved Him ever since I learned about the creation story in the picture book Bible, and learned that He'd thought up all that then became something real, even the naughty sparrow and the silly goose. From my earliest days, He always helped me find my constantly lost hair clips and other things; when I asked Him, I remembered where I had to look.

But I never had confidence in Jesus's ability to have the same imagination and humor as God; I did not have a relationship to him. "What can I do about that?" I asked Molt. "You don't want to force anything, just make yourself wide!" I was determined to make myself "wide." "Visit us for Easter on your way to the kindergarten teacher seminar!"[3] "But that's soooo long till then!" "Then write and let me know how things are progressing!" Yes, I would write to him.

While talking in the hallway, I heard my father quietly opening the door to his study. For him it must have been quite un-matter of fact how much I'd changed since the first two happy days.

We took Molt to the island railway, Armgard and I, and now it even seemed better to me that he was leaving. I needed some quiet for my new development. "Write!" he repeated as the train began to move.

One year later, I was released from Bethel — stamped as an "incurably mentally ill woman." I often asked myself in the following years what the reason for this breakdown was as just five weeks after these events, my psychosis had broken open. Had doubting the "pastor-focused church" pulled the ground out from under my feet? Not just my father but both grandfathers and three uncles were pastors. We lived in this tradition. It seemed to me with Molt, however, that the Christian faith was not based on something passed down, but something experienced directly. He had similarly gleaned his knowl-

3 At this point, Buck had begun training to become a kindergarten teacher.

edge by himself; while with us being educated was, like our faith, a tradition. He had once been a blue-collar worker, he had told us, and he actually wanted to become a poet. That impressed me deeply. Had I sensed through Molt that "being a Christian" demanded more than the root-ball of tradition and the childlike comfort of being in God's presence — that something else had to be added like a spontaneous rain shower to get the roots to grow? My father was more concerned with God as the "father," who for him was the "father full of holy, sternly guiding love," than with Jesus. I had no idea what "holy" love was and "sternly guiding" love must have reminded me what my father's love for me was; both expressions were foreign to me.

Had I realized how much I liked Molt that night by the ocean, how much I needed him and how painful the feeling was to have to live without him? Armgard seemed much less impressed although she had heard the same words. Later on, I would frequently be more unhappily than happily in love, but never again would the ground be pulled away from under my feet like that.

Could he have still elicited such breakdowns if he had been a balanced person? Or was it this conflict within himself, the inner tension, that he gave off, the questioning himself, that ruptured my self-satisfaction? Since Paul, people like him — those who did not quite accept themselves — had exercised a transformative effect on others.

A lot of things probably came together. But I must have had the wish to experience something directly earlier. Because when Father wrote to me in the women's school in 1934 that he was asking to be moved to the island, I had answered that by the sea one must be closer to God. But I was hardly thinking about Jesus at the time.

Once Molt had left, I also wondered whether everything could go back to how it was, whether I could let everything that had been broken up so painfully simply pull itself together again. But I felt that was a retreat into an outdated mode of being that couldn't be fulfilled anymore. I especially loved a poem by Rilke at that time, "The Man Watching," which reads:

> I can tell by the way the trees beat,
> after so many dull days, on my worried windowpanes
> that a storm is coming,
> and I hear the far-off fields say things
> I can't bear without a friend,
> I can't love without a sister.
> The storm, the shifter of shapes, drives on
> across the woods and across time,
> and the world looks as if it had no age:
> the landscape, like a line in the psalm book,
> is seriousness and weight and eternity.[4]

In my apron pocket I carried a small New Testament which I read while doing housework. Because I wanted to grow closer to Jesus. Other times, I would dance my made-up dances outside by the light of the moon. Only now had I begun to feel the full force of puberty. Previously, I had felt unified; now I felt split into a stormy and a mild being, one more male and one female.

I looked for a relationship with Jesus in vain. You just don't feel any guilt, I told myself, and that is why Jesus as the savior from guilt cannot mean much. I listed all my faults and weaknesses in order to fall into the Savior's arms, pushed by the weight of my guilt; having arrived at the last faults, I had already forgotten the first ones. Only three times in my life had I experienced guilt for any longer period of time. The first time, as a child, was when I washed a baby doll with eau de cologne instead of water and realized, full of grief, I would never be able to love

4 Rainer Maria Rilke, *Selected Poems of Rainer Maria Rilke*, trans. Robert Bly (New York: Harper and Row, 1981), 105.

her the way I had because she had three white spots on her red cheeks. The second time I had yelled loudly at my little sister because the kite we constructed from packing paper with Father wouldn't fly; yelling angrily against the wind, I accused her of always placing the tail incorrectly. My older brother descended from the dunes and found my behavior unspeakably bad. I cannot remember ever again being so boundlessly furious. The third time I was still a child, and my sister and I were spending summer break with relatives in the country.

"She gets preferential treatment at home," I told my younger half-cousins, as we sat in the grass and exchanged family stories. "What is 'preferential treatment'?" they wanted to know; they did not know the expression. I explained the word and they decided that their younger sister was also receiving preferential treatment. For years I was full of deep reproach for myself as I never was since. Because surely, I had made them aware of their own disadvantage with that thoughtless word and I knew most of all how it felt to feel discriminated against. In turn, I hardly felt guilty about lies. The adults with all their "no's" forced one to lie because if one could say anything one wanted to, one would not need to lie.

All of that was a long time ago and did not help me any further. Friedrich Lienhard's diary finally gave me the idea that Jesus could also be my savior from deathly fear.[5] I would imagine a hidden murderer was lurking in a dark corner of the hallway or basement and tried to attack me. But even that was in vain; I could barely imagine the shape of the murderer or the sense of deathly fear.

But even if I could have felt guilt—I basically had no idea about the lesson of redemption and guilt. Why should God be less loving than human parents who could

5 Friedrich Lienhard, *Thüringer Tagebüch* (Stuttgart: Verlag von Greiner und Pfeiffer, 1903).

forgive their children without demanding sacrifices and faith? To the present day it still makes no sense to me.

After four weeks of painful attempts at building a relationship with Jesus, I experienced a change. For a week, right after waking up in the morning, something about the message of Christianity I hadn't understood before would make sense. I thought of these morning thoughts as "epiphanies," and for the first time, I believed I understood what Jesus meant by the inner voice, the freedom of conscience, and the words, "If you do not become like the children...."[6] Letting oneself be led was the important thing. I had never before had epiphanies. It is my will not to want something anymore but to let you lead me, I decided. I was happy about this unexpected gift, and it was with this feeling of an entirely new beginning that I wrote to Molt.

I had not succeeded in experiencing Jesus as the redeemer from guilt. But now, when I thought I was experiencing him turning toward me, I really had issues with aspects of myself. I felt the need to free myself from that by writing to Molt. The letter would be a confession, I wrote, and told him how grateful I was that he'd started this process I was experiencing. I was probably even happy to experience a guilty conscience, the way he did, and able to be mad at myself. "I could slap my face on account of my superficiality, labeling people as likable and not likable," I wrote. "The first time I saw you I had no idea what to make of you. But I did not find you likable at all."

For a week, I continued writing this letter using the morning "epiphanies." I only realized much later that I had lost all sense of shame and tact right from the start. My initial childish aversion to Molt, to whom I now felt drawn so strongly, of all people seemed comical to me. I searched for a drastic way to express the comical in this,

6 Cf. Matthew 18:3.

talked of a deaconess I could have spit at because I found her unnatural and added, "With you, I would have waited until I had gotten more because one cannot simply pass you by." And I seriously thought that Molt would also be able to "laugh about that"—the idea that my drastic thoughts could hurt his feelings didn't even occur to me. Finally, I said: "How could I have been so stupid!" I also tried to give him advice. Because Molt could suddenly look so very withdrawn, I wrote: "We must stand steadily on this earth." I was thinking about Walter Flex's *A Wanderer between Two Worlds,*[7] even though I had not read the book. I now thought I had the same feelings as Molt.

It turned into a long letter. A few times, I had the feeling I was savaging myself with this altogether-too-thorough a housecleaning. But I had to avail myself of this opportunity in order not to let it pass me by again. Because I thought of the breakdown as something necessary. Even as a child, the image of the Sower had impressed me very much. On what sort of ground would the seeds fall in my case? I was not too sure whether it might not be suffocated by the weeds.

I also began to doubt my choice of a future career. Was being a kindergarten teacher really right for me? In the women's school I had written a very skeptical essay about education: the children were the lively and imaginative ones while the adults were at risk of being paralyzed by their ideas of order and cleanliness. The essay was not received well; my view of the adults was too pessimistic, I was told. So I wrote to Molt: "Children are much better at raising themselves."

One morning of this week, I realized abruptly that we all wear masks. We are not the way we are but instead

7 Walter Flex, *Der Wanderer zwischen beiden Welten: Ein Kriegserlebnis* (Munich: Beck, 1916), translated into English as *The Wanderer between the Two Worlds: An Experience of War,* trans. Brian Murdoch (London: Rott Publishing, 2014).

the way we think we must be. "Why don't we tear the masks from our faces?" I wrote. "Why are we cramped when we could be natural and beautiful?" The thought that Molt might include himself in this did not occur to me. Because he had moved something in me for that very reason — he showed his feelings, while I had suppressed my feelings from earliest childhood on around not being favored.

While singing I now also wanted something more primal. "The canon of songs cannot fulfill us anymore," I wrote. "Everyone should have their own songs." The song movement had unearthed the old folksongs again. These were wonderful, naive stories about the little golden ring that falls on the girl's foot, and about the farmer who harnesses the cute horses in the month of March; the melodies were narrative, sometimes dancelike and bouncy. But we also sang a fifteenth-century hymn, and it was different from all the other songs. The hymn did not tell a story but was dedicated to a soaring feeling of inner movement and allowed one to feel a great space that corresponded with the ocean, all while breathing and singing. That was what I imagined one's own songs to be like. Later, I made up melodies to the poems of Rilke and other poets.

The first morning of the next week — it was March 1, 1936 — three sentences overcame me with such force that I was nearly pressed to the ground. I was in the laundry room preparing the big laundry load and had just taken pleasure in seeing the pink morning clouds. I heard a voice: a knowing came over me like the epiphanies of the previous week, just much stronger and more forcefully: a monstrous war is coming; I am the "bride of Christ"; someday I will have something to say, and the words will bring themselves forth.[8]

8 Psychologist Thomas Bock, who developed and practiced the trialogue model with Buck, believed this referred to her important

I was so startled that I cried out loudly. I ran to my parents in great excitement and told them what had just happened to me.

We were sitting in Father's study. He tried to calm me down: there would be no war. Then he pulled the Concordance out of his bookcase and explained to me that the "bride of Christ" was an expression for the "community of the holy." Regarding the third sentence, I was informed that young girls did not yet have anything to say. I agreed with him. I would not have known what else to say but that war was on its way. But "is coming," the voice had said, not now.

My mother thought the best thing to do was to dig into the housework. That was not an answer to my shocking experience, but I could understand Mother's frightened defense.

My father's words calmed me, but I could not believe them. Because these couldn't have been my thoughts; they were utterly different from my customary way of thinking and had overcome me as if by force, in the form of epiphanies. How could I have generated the thought of an approaching terrible war when I was hardly interested in politics or history?

Only once during my school time do I remember a historic event having a real impact on me, and I don't think it was even addressed during our lessons. Those were the events around April 1917 when Erich Ludendorff[9] had Lenin, who was living in Switzerland, brought behind the Russian front in a sealed train to break the Russian will to fight by encouraging a revolution. In a poem — it was my first — I expressed my worry that one day, like a boomerang, we would get back the communism Ludendorff had sent the Russians.

speech to a group at the World Psychiatric Association.

9 Erich Ludendorff was a German general, politician, and military theorist.

This event occupied me, and it seemed obvious for me to discuss this with Father since he was very interested in politics and history. But it was hard for me to overcome my shyness. I cannot remember a single real conversation with my father — except for the one preceding confirmation with his confirmation candidates, of which I was one. At the time I felt my relationship with God was too childish, but he said it was perfect that way.

Why didn't my parents ask me what had preceded these initial startling defense reactions? I never understood that. Because these experiences don't happen out of the blue without any preparation. For someone to suddenly be overcome with the sense that war is on the horizon isn't that uncommon, because even animals can sense when a catastrophe or death is pending. But the idea of being the "bride of Christ" was unthinkable without some kind of backstory. In the middle of my dismay and perplexity it would have been such a relief to talk about everything with my parents.

That my mother considered housework, which was my chore, more important than what had overwhelmed me probably was in keeping. Nothing has changed since then in that respect: the individual's work is considered more important than what moves them or what they feel. Maybe that is why Jesus's death on the cross is more important to Christians than what was obviously more important to Jesus: resurrection of the spirit. The redemptive act on the cross, which is how his death is interpreted, was Jesus's work for us. But what the spirit is which, according to Paul, "leads the children of God," how this spirit is experienced and what resurrection of the spirit means, no pastor is able to explain.

Only Molt could help me now because he had triggered this development in me. He was the only one I could trust not to think my "epiphanies" were a mistake emanating from me. My parents were glad that I wanted to ask Molt. The day before my mother had found me writing my letter. "Don't write such a long letter to him!" she said. "At least come down and sit in the warmth!" The way she said it egged on my resistance. Father had been like that as well. When I told him I wanted to interrupt the trip to the kindergarten teachers' seminar in order to visit Molt and his wife, he felt it was totally inappropriate. "You can't stay in a married man's house!" "Why not?" I asked right back. "He invited me." The conventional moralistic ideas of my parents did not apply to my relationship with Molt, I found.

But now, most of all, the "terrible war" had to be stopped. I believed it was looming right in front of us. There had to be something to stop it. And I found a way.

"I remembered something terrible today," I wrote at the end of the letter. "I hardly have the courage to write this to you because you must think I am going crazy or becoming a megalomaniac. First it was just a wish and now I am certain: that people should all become Christians. And that it happens right before the start of a terrible war, which would then not be necessary anymore. You, your wife, and I have to tell the others."

I did not write anything about the force of the attack in the early morning. I probably thought he would certainly think I was crazy if I said anything about it.

"Should you think all of this is nonsense, then please write back immediately. If you don't think it is nonsense, then please come! It would be much better if it were nonsense. My father wants me to eat Promonta[10] for my nerves. My mother thinks I should put all my heart into housework.—I so look forward to Easter when I will be with you. I am not allowed to leave until the Tuesday after Easter and the seminar actually begins on Wednesday. But one or two days more or less won't matter."

I mailed the letter with express courier. "Did you also write on there: 'no night delivery'?" Mother asked with

10 Promonta was a liver extract used in the 1930s for anemia.

concern. That still existed back then. Of course, I had forgotten to.

Exhausted, I went to bed. Not just the threatening war scared me, I was also everything but happy to be the "bride of Christ." Someday, I wanted to have a real husband. But in bed I was able to think everything through again in peace. And I realized that the idea of being the "bride of Christ" was not nonsense. It had to do with the development of my personal nature. I imagined what, realistically, being the bride of Jesus could be like. I would bore him terribly, if I tried to copy him and who he had originally been, by getting over my own nature. And I remembered that important men like Goethe[11] had chosen unimportant but natural women.

That was a relief. I just had to become myself; all the tiring efforts of the last weeks to become something other than what I was were completely unnecessary. I would have constantly fought with my inferiority complex about things I thought Molt might be feeling.

My first reaction to this liberation was to get out my oldest sister's gramophone and records. We looked down on *hits*. I turned up the volume all the way and opened both windows. Alarmed, my father came upstairs. "Hits from a pastor's house!" "Hits are fine," I reassured him. I had to shut the windows.

Then I thought about what to do as the "bride of Christ" and started to create a children's paradise. I sat in a booth at the heavenly fair and demonstrated fantastical clockworks to the wide-eyed children. Children's games would suit me better than Jesus, who showed more of a spirit of joy than amusement. It seemed the saints were also less interested in fun and games.

Playing with the psychotic ideas which broke through from the unconscious could be important and helpful. One opens up to them, creates a relationship with them,

11 Johann Wolfgang von Goethe was a German polymath and writer.

gets to know them more closely, and dedicates internal action to them. This way they do not just lose some of their unfamiliarity; it is also easier to let go of them if one has played them through in all directions and has manifested them in one's fantasy. When a psychotic idea has hardened, then there probably was not enough opportunity to play it out in one's fantasy. The psychiatrist should encourage such playful fantasies rather than fighting them. That is why the breaking in of the otherwise unconscious was a consequential experience for me.

In the language of symbols, the psychotic ideas showed me the way to my true self. I was not able to see that clearly back then. I had not recognized yet that my "epiphanies" had broken through from my unconscious. In Bethel, a second "bride of Christ" was admitted after me. If she'd been helped to understand that the unconscious idea that broke through was a symbol of the development of her singular, God-given nature, she could have developed that idea. Being stamped as an "incurable insane woman," whose experiences are only considered in physical terms and so are useless, instead strengthens the doubt of one's own nature and thus paralyzes one's inner development. This doubt inevitably leads to ever new breaks because to be devalued thus as a human being, and forced into inner isolation, creates a need for the psychotic experiences in which one at least feels accepted by God.

Something else had changed for me. A driving force I had not known previously had erupted in me and I noticed it in even the most quotidian things. When cooking, for example, I used to have to use a cookbook because I couldn't memorize recipes. Now I just let my hands do the work, grabbing whichever ingredients in whatever amount, and my food tasted better than usual. With each of my breaks this instinct was released and the certainty that I could rely on my impulses had something liberating after the deep insecurity of the stigma as a "mentally ill woman."

I waited for Molt's response. My parents did, too. If he had realized how urgent my request was to answer immediately, how desperately I needed reassurance from him that everything was nonsense, then he would probably have sent a brief, quick card. Perhaps it was that the fear of a war on the horizon really seemed nonsensical to him; he, at least, did not want to participate in a general Christianization to hinder the war. Instead, a letter arrived ten days later from the moor. When he thought of our island, he tended to feel guilty, Molt wrote. "Because I assume you have very much been awaiting an answer from me. But you know that good things take their time and I want to respond to your comprehensive letter with a good one." First, he addressed my doubts about becoming a kindergarten teacher, and then responded to my plan of stopping the war: "So often we believe there is a big plan for us. But the greatest thing is to be true to the small things. What that means? We all exist in relationship to other human beings. You in your family, me in mine. That results in tasks that must be accomplished even if it is housework or the like."

That was supposed to be the answer? I felt that with loyalty to the small things, one could not stop a war.

If I'd written of the amount of force with which these three sentences overcame me in the laundry room, he might have realized I couldn't accept that these ideas originated within me. He had advised me to create "space within myself," which could really only mean to create space for something to flow into me. It seemed possible to me that he knew experiences like the ones Rilke expressed in his poem "The Man Watching." Had I now experienced something similar? The idea that this could be "insane" first dawned on me as I spoke with my parents. At the time, they thought of it more as a kind of youthful over-exertion. My father decided I had to take Promonta and got some at the pharmacy that very same morning.

Father came upstairs to see me. "What did he write?" I was lying in bed. The ease with which I had begun to set up the children's heaven was not meant to last. I was getting more and more worried about the thought of the pending war. And Molt's long silence intensified that. I interpreted it as a confirmation of my epiphanies, for if Molt had thought they were nonsense then surely he would have written back immediately. I gave Father the letter.

"How well he describes and poetically he writes about this!" He read the words following the beginning out loud. "We walk out into the heath together. And you tell me so much about yourself and your thoughts. The fog settles in big swaths over the heather and the juniper looks like a small, crippled man who shakes his fists menacingly...."

"He means himself with that," I said. "He is passionate and suffers from it!" Molt sent his regards to "blood brother Bello." I didn't quite know what to make of his response, but I lost myself more and more in the image of the juniper with raised fists on the lonely heath. It gave rise to the wildest assumptions. The only thought I did not have, which was so obvious, was that I could have hurt his feelings and the menacing juniper fists were his reaction to that. I felt beat up. In the afternoon, Father came upstairs again. I pretended to be sleeping. He stroked my hair and left again.

The next time he came upstairs, I randomly explained to him that the mother of the illegitimate child in the neighborhood, who insisted on not naming the father, was not at all as "bad" as he'd said. On the contrary, one had to admire her, and I wished I could act the way she had. But unfortunately, I wasn't far along enough yet for that. I had thought about whether I could do that: to have an illegitimate child, to take the stain of the adulteress upon myself, and to refuse to name the man in order to spare him the trouble. Was my love for Molt deep enough for that? As deep as this woman's from the neighborhood, whom I considered anything but "bad?" I was convinced I couldn't do what she did.

Mother came upstairs. "Do you have children?" Father had asked Molt. No, he had said, not yet, but he hoped there would be some. Of the three years he had been married, he had only been home a quarter of a year.

I had put my favorite doll on the blanket at the foot of my bed. "Molt will have a daughter, my godchild," I now told Mother. "She will get my doll." Mother listened to me, shaking her head and worried.

Later there was a second letter. Molt asked whether I had received his first one? He had not yet received a response. He reported on his church music trips. His choir was now singing a passion by Heinrich Schütz—with the hymn "Jesus, your passion now I'll think about" they entered the church. He wrote about the deep joy that filled him when he stood in front of his choir. These were very simple people who had worked their way into the music with such love, with diligence, and with patience, that it was a joy to be around.

In the first days of April, Mother took me to see a doctor in her native town. He was not a psychiatrist; it would have been much too risky to visit a psychiatrist during the Nazi period. I gave him the little notebook in which I had written my epiphanies. "I can't read it," the doctor said. "You have to read it to me." Already impatient, he handed me the notebook. Reading out loud was anything but pleasant to me, because reading out loud made it clear to me that my forms of expression were completely my own. Therefore, only the content of the ideas could have been supplied to me.

Then I begged the doctor to go see Hitler with me so we could warn him about the war. Because the idea of the pending war worried me ever more deeply, and three-and-a-half years later war really did start. "I can't just leave my practice," he answered. He placed me behind a screening device as if he could recognize my spirit in the X-ray.

We walked through the city parks, my mother, my oldest sister—she was going to vocational school in the doctor's town—and I. A blooming forsythia — I stood still in front of it as if it were a miracle. What a magical spirit that had imagined the flowers, the shrubs and trees, and this blossoming bush! Since the morning in the laundry room, my moods had gone back and forth between fear and happiness, between the deep worry about the pending war, and the joy-bringing feeling of being loved by this spirit, of knowing I was being led.

I called Molt from the hospital. In the middle of peeling an orange I felt compelled to. "We are here in A." "Yes?" "We saw the doctor today. I told him what was going to happen. But he didn't believe me." "Did you receive both of my letters?" "Yes, but they did not impress me at all." "Why not?" "Your premise is completely wrong. That's not so bad." "What's not so bad?"

Right, how could I have explained this to him? How could I have told him that he had no reason to suffer from himself? That feelings couldn't be anything negative but that only the lack of feelings was bad?

"What have you been up to?" I asked him. He had sung more passions with his choir. Singing! When we had to stop a war! "You must come immediately!"

"Of course I won't come," Molt said. "I don't know what you want from me. May I please speak with your mother?" "Yes, but you can't make it sound too bad!" "I won't make it sound bad at all." "But you'll come!" I said it like a command.

I got my mother. Basically, I found it terrible that she dragged me to the doctor. That she degraded as sick what I experienced as God's guidance. I was not motivated to ask her afterwards whether Molt was coming. She had certainly not encouraged him to do so. It was surely just unpleasant for her that I had called him. She had no idea of my breakdown after the second song evening. And if he had come after all? I probably would not have been open to his arguments and would have insisted that only he and I had to warn Hitler about the "terrible" war.

I still could not believe that his "Of course I won't come; I don't know what you want from me" should have been his last words. Back on our island, I went straight to the airport the next day—and asked whether a married couple had arrived. "No." I described Molt and his wife. "No, they did not arrive."

How was the war to be stopped now?

And then the miracle on the moor happened, my rebirth, then the room with bars in the mainland hospital. On the drive to Bethel—because that is where they took me, but I did not know that—I saw Molt one more time. Already dazed from the injection, I read a sign: Halle. Where are we? shot through my mind—Halle is situated on the Saale.[12] It was the Westphalian Halle, right before Bielefeld. At a crossing in the city, I saw Molt sitting in a dark car. He looked grim and desperate—a projection of my own desperation as I later realized. Someone I didn't know sat next to him at the wheel and his stiff hat looked as if it had been pushed back from his bare forehead. He was just leaning his head back and laughing.

12 The Saale is a German river and tributary of the Elbe.

3

Hell amidst Bible Quotes

In Bethel I was given a bed in a communal sleeping hall that was part of the "agitated ward." This ward was in a house "for nervous and mood disorders": that is what it was called back then. A stout deaconess approached my bed. She brought a little glass with a bitter-smelling liquid. It was paraldehyde, which I would have to drink so often moving forward. Poison! I thought right away. I had come from the island full of trust, but in the meantime I'd found out that nobody cared about my best interests. I was being fought against.

I fell out of the bed, grabbed the vase with the Easter flowers from the little ward table and drank all of it to dilute the poison with water. Then I jumped on a bench near the window and from there onto the windowsill, tried in vain to push myself through the narrow opening of the barely open window, and yelled loudly for help.

The next morning, I experienced the second doctor's visit in this eerie house. I had received for my second breakfast an orange from which a bad piece had been cut out. "Have we already been gnawed on?" the head physician asked and looked at the hole in the piece of fruit. I asked in return whether everyone here had syphilis. "How did you know that?" was his answer. "From the home economics dictionary." He shook his head. "From the home economics dictionary!"

These words of welcome were to be the longest medical conversation during the entire nine months of what was to be my ward time in Bethel.

I had drawn my education from the home economics dictionary; it was to remain accordingly incomplete. My suspicion that I would find syphilis here had reasons. The previous evening the head ward nurse had wished me "good night" and added: "Sleep well into your wedding night!" My epiphany of being the "bride of Christ" had probably led to her ridiculous wish. Teasing like this is a sport among the nursing personnel but it is everything but harmless for us patients. The ward, especially the first time, is much too scary for us to understand such jokes.

In Gedat's book *A Christian Experiences the Problems of the World*,[1] which at the time was considered sensational, I had found out about the existence of brothels a few months prior. If I was to spend my "wedding night" here, then this foreign house in which I was being held like a prisoner and numbed with poison could only be a brothel. This reasoning was absolutely logical for me. The stories about men that another patient told the nurses only reinforced my thinking. During the first weeks in this ward the idea that the ward nurse wanted to hook me up with the devil was sheer torture.

Half the night I gazed fearfully at the glass door through which the men were going to enter. How could I protect myself from them? But eventually sleep got the better of me. I fought sleep for a long time because if I were to fall asleep, I would be a helpless victim of the men. Finally, I had an idea how to save myself: they would recoil from stench. When the nurse pulled back the covers in the morning, she found the mess.

1 Gustav Adolf Gedat, *Ein Christ erlebt die Probleme der Welt: Versuch einer volkstümlichen Einführung in das Weltgeschehen unserer Tage* (Stuttgart: J.F. Steinkopf, 1934).

The next morning, she found the same thing in my bed. That set the tone for our relationship: Nurse Y thought that I wanted to make her mad. But I only wanted to protect myself. From that point on I noticed I was not in a brothel. The house was even more different than I'd thought and couldn't be understood. My fellow sufferers had in fact not caught syphilis; there had to be other reasons why some of them looked so odd.

Here too, no explanation was provided. Nobody told us why we were here and why we were being held prisoner. I now put all my attention and intelligence into finding out what kind of a house this was. It couldn't be a hospital because there were no medical exams, no rounds, and no treatments. I had wound up in a static world: everything was sterile. We were forced to do nothing and had to stay in bed although we were physically healthy. That led to the wildest fears and notions for me.

Everything I found obvious at home, even after my psychotic break, was taken away from me here; the freedom to move and to act, the words one exchanged while doing so, and the feeling of equality. As powerless, guarded women we stood here opposite our guards who could move about freely. Certainly, I had also become an object of worry for my parents since the unsettling event that morning in the laundry room. I heard them talk about me full of worry, while my worry focused on the great war that I thought would be upon us momentarily. It also seemed unnatural to me that they knew nothing of the restless weeks prior to this dramatic event and my previous breakdown, nor what I had experienced as a logical development in that context, except the three confusing sentences. Nonetheless, they had remained my partners.

When my mother came upstairs with her down blanket the evening before April 9, to sleep in the bed next to mine, I would not have any of it. I found her worry completely unnecessary. "Let's stop that right now!" I said and wouldn't let her in. This rejection must have hurt her deeply because I always had a close relationship with her, even if we did not speak much. I think she went back down to my father crying. He came upstairs beside himself.

"An eye that scorns obeying father and mother should be pecked by the ravens by the stream and eaten by the young eagles"[2] he threw my way as a response. Scared, I stared at my father in his Old Testament anger. And apparently, he even scared himself because immediately, he gave me a desperate kiss. I knew it was all a result of my parents' worry for me. Here at Bethel, however, I was only an observed object not worth offering a question or an answer.

A human being can hardly be degraded more. The doctors and nurses who know nothing and want to know nothing about the history and the contextual meaning of the psychosis, and think everything is just a meaningless side effect of a physical disease, probably never think about how they degrade and devalue us. As long as they don't talk to us, they cannot know anything about us.

Was I supposed to recant what I had experienced? Is that what they wanted? Did the old authoritarian demand of the church to recognize only what fit their ideas of God's path for humans, and keep people from questioning their role as mediators, present itself in a new form of resistance, one that was more contemporary than medieval methods? I swore that I would never exchange what I had experienced as God's guidance for the "true Christianity" that was being modeled here. Following each narcotic injection and each little glass of paraldehyde I was given, I insisted to Nurse Y. that none of this would ever change my mind, and I repeated this until I passed out.

On the green wall across from me painted in large letters was Jesus's quote: "Come to me, all you who are weary

2 Proverbs 30:17.

and burdened, and I will give you rest."[3] Refresh—with long baths and wet wraps, with cold water showers on the head, with narcotic injections and paraldehyde. That was absurd and incomprehensible. I had to think of God calling the devil "the father of lies." And then something happened that made an indelible impression on me. Frau Pastor H. was cleaning the hall dressed in the blue-striped ward uniform and talking to herself. Maybe the tone was aggressive and maybe she looked at Nurse Y. Regardless, the squat deaconess suddenly grabbed the Frau Pastor's long hair, pulled her down to the ground, and dragged her across the floor by her hair. She passed the Bible quote going into the bathroom. Like a strong field horse in front of the plow she looked at us—an unforgettable image of brutal violence and unprotected impotence.

Decades have passed since then and still that image is embedded in my mind's eye as if it happened yesterday. And that is probably how all of us affected ones feel who have had the most harrowing experiences in our asylums—possibly in Christian asylums with Bible quotes on the walls. If that is supposed to be spiritual health—it could not convince us. We learned to fear this type of "spiritual health."

Nurse G., the second-in-command ward nurse, helped Nurse Y. She always seemed unfulfilled, almost unhappy, to me, and as the only independent nurse aside from the two friendly young night nurses, Margarete and Charlotte, it probably wasn't easy for her among the deaconesses. Together they pushed the patient's head under the cold-water faucet. Then Nurse Y. threw a towel her way: "There, dry yourself off again!"

Deep fears and an increasing confusion filled me. Why had my parents not told me any of this? They had sent me here so they must have been in the know. Following

3 Matthew 11:28. In German, the second phrase is rendered with "Ich will Euch erquicken," literally "I will refresh you."

rounds, I was put in the duration bath. A sailcloth was pulled over the tub, only the head was free; a stiff collar came around the neck. Now fear overcame me, they wanted to give me a Satan's child by magic. Close all holes so that the water can't penetrate you, I told myself. I even held my belly button closed just in case, although it wasn't easy to cover three body openings with two hands—and that for twenty-three hours till the next morning. Because that's how long I had to stay in the duration bath. During the night, the nice young night nurse filled the bath with warm water using a faucet that had been attached to the tub from the outside, and she did it in such a knowing way, as if it was the most natural thing in the world that I should be lying in a bathtub at night rather than a bed. Completely exhausted and beaten, run down from the lack of sleep and the immobility of the locked-in neck, I climbed out of the tub the next day. And fear of a repetition of this torturous procedure made me keep quiet for quite some time.

The less I understood the nature of this imprisonment the greater my fear grew. Finally, I asked to be put into the little separate room. Because I didn't want to have to constantly see the "calming techniques" being used in the hall. Here I now experienced the "wet pack": I was wrapped into wet, cold cloths so tightly that I couldn't move anymore. My body warmth made the cloths first warm and then hot. I screamed with indignation against this senseless torture. In reports from Soviet special institutions for dissidents, the tying up with wet cloths, which tighten around the body as they dry, is considered the most terrible form of torture. It surely was even more gruesome in the Soviet institution, but what I experienced was bad enough. It felt to me like an ordeal and a punishment, and that it happened under Bible quotes heightened my fear and confusion even more. As a "calming technique" this wet pack would have been just as useless for a healthy person.

This house became ever scarier, and I wanted to have as little as possible of it around me. I demanded that the other beds and my own bed space be pushed out. I had the pictures and the framed Bible quotes taken from the walls. The house mother did it herself. I only kept my mattress. But the mattress scared me as well because it was part of the house. That why I painted it and the inner door — now the only movable objects in the room — with a cross of feces. I covered the entire surface with it; it was the only way I could protect myself from what felt to me like hell under Bible quotes.

I spent about ten days in deep fear such as I had never experienced before and never would again. To get my fear under control, I would sing "God is a mighty stronghold" for hours with the third verse, "And if the world were full of devils and wanted to engulf us...." I did not eat or drink anymore because nothing of this scary house was to penetrate me. I was force-fed through a tube in my nose.

The coarse gray smock I was dressed in was a special torment. It was fastened in the back by the collar. That I had to wear something on my body from this house intensified my fear of being subjugated. Because the material was too thick to tear, I pulled my arms out of the sleeves of the smock and turned it constantly and slowly around me so that it never had to touch me too long. In the evening, after I had received a sedative injection and felt myself passing out, I pulled out a strand of hair and put it between myself and the clasp on the collar to protect myself from the touch of the smock, and thus from the power of the house. I felt the effects here of an old magical idea, one found in fairytales and myths. This idea has lasted into our time with the saying, "Whose clothing one wears, that's whose servant one is."

The head physician was making his rounds. He sat next to me on the mattress on the floor and took me into his arms. "But you are my friend!" How could anyone talk about friendship! Did he want to test my reaction? I held him off: "I am not your friend! Don't touch me! I don't belong to you!" The smock I had to wear, the intrusive embrace, the nutrition liquid that entered me by nose — it all roused a deep fear in me, in the power of this scary house, to be a victim of the devil's power.

After about ten days I knocked at the door that had a peephole and asked for nine oranges. But I only received two — the first meal I ate again. Why it had to be nine exactly I don't remember. I was lying in my bed in the group hall again. The beech forest behind the high wall of the ward garden had turned green again in the meantime; previously the trees had still been bare.

These almost inhuman fears, triggered by a senseless treatment that assaults instead of helping, were a penetrating experience and have remained important to me to the present. They taught me, physically, that it is not faith that is the deciding factor, witnessed by the quotes on walls and daily mottos, but rather the will to communicate and imagination. Only if one acknowledges a mentally ill person's humanity, recognizes their situation, and respects their feelings, can one help them.

Nurse Y. approached my bed: What did I want to have for lunch. I didn't know. "Perhaps a little dove?" She seemed to want to make me strong again. But not a little dove, no! I wouldn't eat it! How can you offer me a dove as a meal — the symbol of the Holy Ghost!

In vain I tried to find out why we were here. No conversation, no work, no examination or treatment — it remained completely incomprehensible. Every morning there were rounds. In single file they entered the hall: the chief physician at the front, who of all of them still seemed the most natural and so most trustworthy, followed by the three assistant physicians and finally the house mother. One morning, the chief physician and the female assistant physician headed straight toward me. It seemed arranged. Both of them placed themselves at the head of my bed, he to the right, she to the left, but not facing me, rather the center of the hall. Like guard soldiers or guardian angels, I thought. The house mother stood at the foot of the bed. I lay on the flat bed leaning on my elbows, shook my head, and laughed. What was this all about? Did they want to test my reaction again? "It is all much more serious than you think," the assistant physician said. Why didn't she tell me what was more serious?

The hall was painted light green, five to six white steel tube beds stood on each of the long sides of the room. The wide glass door to the bathroom with toilet and two bathtubs was always open. The faucets of the sinks were unlocked with a latchkey only in the morning; to open them in the evening for washing and brushing teeth apparently involved too much work. To the right of the bathroom there was a small separate room with a peephole in the door. These three rooms — actually the hall and the bathroom were just one — were our entire living area. It was only after many weeks when I was finally allowed to get up — some lay in bed the whole time during the eleven weeks I was in this ward — that I saw the space expanded by a porch next to the separate room that had a table and a bench. From here a wide concrete ramp led down to the little ward garden, encircled by a high wall.

The hall was bright. On both the long sides behind the beds there were tall windows one could only open a tiny bit. From my bed, through the window behind me, I could see an almost-square little piece of lawn with a round bed of roses in the middle. A more than six-foot-high chain-link fence separated it from the ward garden. Still, and as if lifeless, this little rose garden was situated in a niche between our "restless" and the adjacent "quiet" ward, surrounded by a fence and walls. One time I saw a nurse picking roses there.

Through the slanted window on the opposite side between the wall with the Jesus quote and a wooden corner bench, I looked out at a gray-yellow boulder. Massive and wide, it rested beside a climbing path, an avenue. Just like the silent rose garden, this boulder seemed enchanted.

Besides myself, there were two other young girls there, Little R. and Little P. — we were all addressed by our surnames with diminutives at the end. Little R., daughter of a doctor from Frankfurt, was a beautiful girl with dark curls. Apparently, she had experienced something similar to me that had shaken her to the core. Her first love, it seemed to me. She could grasp as little as I did what all of this was about. Little P., around twenty-five to twenty-eight years old, was diagonally across from me beside the corner bench and table. Apparently, she'd been here a long time already; she had acclimated. How does one feel, with these innocent, childlike arm and hand movements that she made sitting in bed? I tried these movements out. It was a schematic not a natural movement, I found. Was it a kind of protection? Or a vent in order not to spontaneously jump out of bed and subsequently be punished with the "calming techniques" like we restless ones were? But I myself was constantly circling my right foot in its joint. That attracted the attention of the female assistant physician.

All the stereotypical movements of locked-up institutional patients are the last remaining movement of human beings who have been forced into complete passivity. Even the childlike arm and hand movements P. made could be explained this way. And it actually made more sense to move the arms and hands that had been forced into passivity than to constantly circle a foot that I'd rather have used to get up and walk.

Later a young aristocratic woman joined, Fräulein von W. She had been operated on recently. She kept getting up from bed. What were those peculiar scars that she and Little R. and Little P. had above their vaginas? I asked Nurse Y. "Appendix scars," she explained. Earlier on I'd learned that the appendix was located on the side. Had we been lied to about that as well? Then at some point the second "bride of Christ" was admitted, a woman around thirty.

Our two pastors' wives had not submitted, although they had both been here a long time. Both seemed to be in their forties. Mrs. H., who was dragged into the bath so brutally, I've already mentioned. The fate of the other one is unforgettable for me. I was told that she had five or six children. Prior to the last child her husband had been warned by the doctor: his wife was not to have any more children. But the child was born and since then she had been in the institution. The husband divorced her and remarried because the children needed a mother, after all. She was full of silent bitterness and sometimes banged her head with the shorn hair against the walls of the hall.

Mrs. Pastor H. uttered her protest with her head raised looking up. At first, I thought she was playing "chicken"—just like I had played "galloping horse" in bed, because we had to pass the time doing something. But then I realized that she had to tilt her head and keep it raised like that in order to vent her feelings without being punished; it was her only option. When she spoke to the ceiling nobody felt addressed; keeping her head straight she knew the nurses would feel her protest was directed at them, and they would again have shoved her head under the cold water faucet.

Our two pastors' wives were the only ones on the ward who worked. They washed and polished the floors of the hall and were taken to the kitchen almost daily to prepare the vegetables. The hall was spic and span. A spot would have immediately been noticed. The lacking humanity went unnoticed—except for those of us who were affected.

I lay between two little Marie's. Little Marie G. on the right lay in bed the whole time I was there, almost always strapped in the waist belt made of white stuff. She had a strangely yellow skin color and was already completely gray, although I thought she was only in her thirties, because her green eyes sparkled vividly. Only later was it revealed that Nurse Y. sometimes beat her — on account of her injuries. Years later the assistant doctor from back then, who in the meantime had been promoted to chief physician, told me.

Little Marie to my left seemed completely apathetic and only left behind a weak impression on me. But I will never forget that she once bled from her rectum. The appendix in the middle, one's menses from the rectum — everything here seemed to go against nature.

And then there were four older women there. Mrs. von B. was so emaciated she almost looked like a skeleton and was full of bedsores, although she lay on a rubber ring; she had purulent wounds. Sometimes she swayed out of the separate room in a short nightgown. "My God! My God!" She repeated this high-pitched lament often. The nurses sometimes echoed it. She and another woman died during this time, and I felt as if I was taking part in their death.

Twice I received little packages of beach carnations and other dune flowers from home. Why did they send these wild freedom flowers to my imprisonment? Something to keep me occupied would have been much more needed. I put the flowers on the bed of the old woman across from me. She had brought her high felt slipper holding urine to my bed. Did she also not want to sit on the toilet? I was to sit down on the toilet properly, as was customary, Nurse Y. had warned me. "I'm not supposed to sit on others' toilets, my father told me." The old woman took the flowers and held them in her hand, I think she was happy. Three days later she was dead. The second time I got dune flowers I put them on the bed of the woman with the sores in the separate room. Three days later, she too was dead. You can't put wildflowers on other beds anymore, I told myself, because here they are heralds of death—where only death can be the liberation from an unbearable imprisonment.

There was also an unmarried woman who never said a word, and an old woman who spoke constantly. Not even the duration bath could get her to be silent. "The little and the big minds are the hardest to deal with," the chief physician said as he was leaving. Nurse Y. pulled a pillowcase over the old woman's head, which stuck out of the collar of the sailcloth over the tub. When she finally took off the pillowcase again, the old woman was blue in the face.

And that was supposed to be Bethel? The Bethel for which as children we ate rye bread in order to send Pastor Fritz von Bodelschwingh the saved pennies? He had thanked us with a delightful letter. Was everything completely different from what we had learned?

And how could my parents subject me to this hell? In particular, to do so because of the most important experience of my life, my rebirth! Except for the year at the women's school,[4] I had spent nineteen years with my family. But they didn't care about me, didn't visit me, just sent me dune flowers.

From Mother I got picture postcards, she wrote a few words about visits to family and friends. My siblings didn't write at all. I had no idea that short cards were only allowed once in a while, and that my father was not allowed to see me when he was in the house; he had accompanied my sister to the women's school and tried, on his return, to visit me. My uncle, too, who had been in Bethel for a conference, had not been allowed to visit.

Perhaps, I thought, so-called hell actually was taking place on earth. Because God's actions are only tolerated here on earth when they are part of the past; those who experience hell today are sent to Bethel by their relatives,

4 Buck is referring to her time in kindergarten teacher training.

in order to exorcize it. But I would not let it be exorcized; I was determined.

Bethel as "City of Charity" could, at any rate, only be a lie. What other things could possibly be different from what we had learned? Bethel's answer to the experiences that were fundamental for me shook my worldview as deeply as the moor experience had. If miracles still happen today, I told myself, then the desiccation of the Red Sea through which Moses led his people had been true, too. Could fairytales then possibly be true as well? During afternoon rounds I asked the chief physician, who seemed trustworthy to me, whether he could turn into Molt. Right in the beginning I had explained to the house mother that Molt and his wife were going to come and get me out of here. In the meantime, I had given up this hope but perhaps there was a last chance through a transformation.

The chief physician backed off a little, hesitated for an instant, and then said: "Yes, I can do that." He probably hoped that I would transfer my trust in Molt onto him. Because I noticed his uneasiness answering, I did not have much confidence in his transformation talents. But at least he'd admitted that transformations like the ones in fairytales were even possible. So I could try to regain my freedom through a word that would release the magical spell as it did in fairytales; there didn't seem to be another solution. And the thought wasn't that off, after all, that I had to have landed in a bewitched world whose spell could only be broken when we guessed the magic word and could properly throw the ball back that had been thrown our way. Because this ward was scary and unnatural; instead of conversations, human care, and activities there was only punishment and "calming techniques." And all of this under Jesus quotes that didn't fit at all.

When the morning rounds group left the hall, the chief physician in front, followed by the assistant doctors and the house mother, and last of all the ample Nurse Y., I called in their direction: "The fat tail end is on its way!" Another time I encircled her with the words "You are mine, I am yours," while she beat my back with the iron door handle that was attached to a long leather belt until I couldn't breathe, and I had to let go of her.

"You poor things that you are forced to do this!" I said with honest empathy, because she seemed to me to be under a spell and to really be bewitched. During the closing party of a youth vacation camp by the Baltic Sea, I once played Jorinde in the fairytale play,[5] who with a blue flower turned her Joringel and all the others who'd been transformed into birds and locked in cages back into human beings. If one keeps one's human figure, I told myself, then one perhaps doesn't notice one has been bewitched. Nurse Y. should probably never have been allowed to become a deaconess; it seemed to me that celibacy was not good for her.

Another time, I'd gotten up out of bed, gone over to Little P.'s bed and sat on the frame and told her a dream. She listened attentively and took my wrist in her hands, just like someone who had at first been very mad at me in my dream. "But then he wasn't mad anymore." "No," she said, smiling, "he wasn't mad at you anymore." Nurse Y. interrupted us, took me back to my bed, and tied me up tightly with a belt made of white stuff. Up till then I had only seen that done to very young children; and so I played with my hands in front of my face the way babies do and called, "Mama! Papa!" And I was truly surprised that I once again didn't do the right thing. Nurse Y. scolded I should finally get reasonable. "Get reasonable" — that could only mean to become inhumane; what was modeled as reason here was something I absolutely did not want to adopt.

5 "Jorinde and Joringel" is a fairytale by the Brothers Grimm in which a witch's spells are ended by a magic flower.

It truly was a bewitched world: Nobody struck up a conversation with us, we weren't allowed to talk to each other, no games and no crafts, every initiative stopped, instead only forced measures meant to "calm." Of course, it wasn't Nurse Y.'s fault but that of the directors of the house. Pastor Fritz von Bodelschwingh and the Bethel parish priests should have known that locked-up patients who are only held all day long and stopped from occupying themselves must naturally become restless; they would surely have to with such treatment. And then the artificially induced restlessness is fought against with forced measures! Nowadays this is done with medication, which paralyzes one's natural initiative.

I registered every indication of a change in the nurses attentively and with worry. After all, I didn't have anything else to do. If they were quieter than usual, that could mean it was the stillness that precedes the storm. If Nurse Y. entered the hall in a more agitated way than usual, even that was alarming. Sometimes the atmosphere in the ward was filled with so much unbearable tension only a cloudburst could bring soothing calm. The constant presence of this unsatisfied person who had absolute power to punish us with "calming" measures for the slightest sign of life put us in a state of constant tension and fearful restlessness. Only Little Marie to my left and Little P. did not seem to be bothered much by this senseless imprisonment. Perhaps they had just been used to it for too long.

Many years later I was talking to the chief physician about Nurse Y. She had been a "witch," the doctor said, and because of her abuse of Little Marie G. she was finally transferred to a general hospital. But for the nurses it must surely have also been depressing to only be allowed to store us. They had not been the ones who invented the duration baths and the "wet wraps," and surely would never have dared to defy the doctors' orders. They apparently didn't have the guts to talk to us because the doctors declared any conversation with us meaningless. And they never experienced healing, because as soon as a patient seemed only temporarily disturbed, she would just be put into a different ward. The nurses were also the victims and carried the burden of the psychiatric dogma of the physically caused and therefore meaningless "endogenous psychosis." And to this day institutions are everywhere where no one talks to the patients about the psychosis experience, to help them understand the positive meaning in it. Instead, they try to break every resistance with numbing psychotropic drugs.

In the following weeks, I had a hallucination that remains unforgettable, but which didn't make sense to me for a long time. During noon nap time I had the impulse to lie under the blanket — even covering my head — and just wait to see what would happen. Nurse Y. approached my bed and patted the top of the blanket. Under her touch a small glowing red spot grew.... It spread until the entire blanket covering me was glowing red and hot. Although I knew I just had to throw back the blanket to let the apparition disappear, I somehow wasn't "allowed" to. I was sweating and prayed under the unbearably red, glowing, and hot blanket until the redeeming moment came and I could throw back the cover. I emerged from under the blanket red like a crab and covered in pimples. I took off my shirt, rubbed myself with spit, and sat down in the sun that was shining on my bed. The redness and pimples disappeared again; they only remained in my armpits and developed into actual boils which finally had to be treated with X-rays. My hair fell out strands at a time.

How was I supposed to understand that? I had experienced the red-hot blanket, had physically felt the heat; my rash, the boils, and the hair loss were incontestably real. Only years after my last break did I find an explanation in Ernst Kretschmer's *Medical Psychology:* "All of the image syntheses which occur in the thinking of the healthy acculturated person on the edge, i.e., on the dark periphery of consciousness behind the abstract, in schizophrenic thinking replace the abstract and become the light focal point of the mental field of vision."[6] So, in its schizophrenic state, abstract thinking turned into symbolic thinking. Kretschmer continues: "A schizophrenic really sees fire and is actually burned, while a healthy person would say: I have feelings of love and thoughts of love."[7] Or such was the case with me: I had the feeling of being in a hell amongst Bible quotes.

When such a visceral experience of thought is simply put down as "pathologic," then we cannot learn to understand our experiences. One imagines "pathologic" refers to something invented, that doesn't exist in reality. The lived symbol, however, is something real; in my case it was so physically real the results needed X-rays to go away.

Why should the physical experience of an internal idea be pathologic? It only proves that mental ideas can change the body and thus refutes the stance that spirit and material are separate entities. The belief in purgatory, which probably leads back to similar experiences, is not considered pathologic. And the stigmata of saints also are not considered pathologic even though the wounds can only have opened through inner imaginative power. That is why they appear in the palm and not at the base of the hand. In reality a crucifixion was only possible at the base of the hand, as is shown by examinations of the Shroud of Turin; in the traditional theory, however, nails burrowed through the palms, and that is how the crucifixion is always represented in art.

I found Kretschmer's explanation helpful even if it only offers speculation. Because it represents an attempt

6 Ernst Kretschmer, *Medizinische Psychologie*, 3rd ed. (Leipzig: Georg Thieme, 1926), 105.

7 Ibid.

at understanding how a physical experience of internal ideas can become possible in the schizophrenic state. And additionally, it showed me that other schizophrenics experience similar things to mine; and so, I felt less alone.

In this ward which was so hermetically cut off from the outside world that no visitor was allowed to enter, symbolic language and symbolic actions had literally run wild. I will give an example of an argument on the symbolic level that schizophrenics have in common. I already mentioned the unmarried woman who never said a word. The opposite of the similarly quiet pastor's wife, who had five or six children, the first woman's attitude toward us younger ones had something hostile. She and I did not like each other. One evening—the ward clock read ten to seven—on my way from the bathroom to my bed, I walked toward the table at which she was sitting, propped both my hands on the tabletop, looked at her, and thought: in ten minutes, at seven o'clock!

But I didn't say anything. The woman accepted my challenge. At seven on the dot, she got up, passed the glass door of the bathroom, and positioned herself with her back to the hall by the right post of the door frame. Then, against her will, she turned toward me three times—I sat up in my bed—and went back to her place. That was it, but from that time on our relationship changed, even if it didn't get better. Until then she had scared me; now I apparently scared her because from then on, she always made a detour around my bed. I had transmitted the time "at seven o'clock" telepathically, but not the rules of the "duel": I hadn't thought about that part at all. That a turning-around-toward-someone counts as an expression of having lost can probably only be found in fairytales and myths these days. There is a sense of that in the story of Orpheus in the underworld and also in Ezekiel's visions of angels; Lot's wife turned into a pillar of salt when she turned around.

I, too, now turn back but in the hope that my report can contribute to a better understanding of the schizophrenic patient.

This close connection of schizophrenics on a common level of symbols dissolves again when we have won back our "thick skin." This suggests the similarity of the changes from normal we experience.

Dr. G., one of the young assistant doctors, said goodbye to us in the hall; he wanted to go on vacation. In the door to the building's annex, he turned around again and saw me sitting in bed holding up both of my index fingers to form a cross. He looked at me in a serious and accusatory way and then disappeared through the door to the ward garden. In the garden wall there was a steel door leading out into the open. Oh, what had I done? To protect myself I had laid a cross made of mortar guides on myself in the hospital basement, and as protection here I had painted a cross on the door and the mattress. But I didn't need to protect myself from Dr. G. and yet I had held the cross against him. Why had he looked at me in such a serious and accusatory way? What if that meant I wished him the cross, that he should be crucified! Deep fear filled me. If only he came back so that I could take it back, reverse what I had done without thinking it through!

He came back. I jumped out of bed, took off my nightgown, and went down on my knees before him: "Forgive me please!" The nurses came over laughing, among them a younger deaconess from the adjacent "quiet ward," who pulled me up, dressed me in a house nightgown, and took me back to my bed. I could have skipped making that gesture. And it had come at such a cost to me. And now to top it off, I had a house nightgown on my body! And I had gone down to my knees, had basically subjugated myself to him!

Pastor H., a man of about forty, went from bed to bed. Aside from the older Pastor K. with Parkinson's disease, he was the only visitor who was allowed in here. At each bedside, he took the patient's hand and with an unnaturally soft voice quoted a Bible verse. As if he couldn't talk with his natural voice and was not allowed to talk to us personally in his own words. When he also recited a verse to me, I couldn't hold back my laughter. Now I thought I knew what the meaning of this city of charity was. His dark eyes got large, pupil and iris floated like islands in the white of his eyeball. With a raised voice he continued to speak beseechingly and now I was laughing loudly. That God's word in this venue, spoken with such an unnatural voice at that, must seem like mockery, was something he couldn't understand.

I was not familiar with this deluge of Bible quotes: biblical house names, Bible quotes on the walls, Bible quotes out of the mouths of both the pastors. At home one read "Wurster's Devotionals" and later the "Words," and on holidays there was lots of singing and music making; my parents looked for practical help in their congregation, but this verbal piety was new to me.

In 1977, I received a calendar from Bethel, *A Hundred Years of a Deacon Institution in Nazareth in Bethel,* and in it I found a saying by Father Bodelschwingh: "Oh, take precious care of those souls who have been put in your care and do not look at them as they are, but see the high cost that has been paid on their behalf!" When I read that I asked myself whether this attitude automatically must lead to replacing natural human care with the quoting of the Bible. The "high cost" could only be referring to Jesus's death, and from this death the entire value of a human life was derived, instead of looking at the individual and respecting them for who they were. And the conversion to Jesus was considered salvation of the soul and not the development of a human's nature as it was given by God, and which can only develop when it's respected. But when the pastors, or those who care for the soul, felt this unworthy caretaking was sufficient and their only task was to provide Bible quotes — then how obvious that the long-term patients had to turn into shriveled souls after years of inactivity!

A terrible suspicion arose inside of me. What if Jesus himself was the charlatan—Jesus, under whose quotes on the wall we were not being "refreshed" but fought against? Could all of this only be a misunderstanding of his teaching? So many prayers for almost two thousand years, so many reaffirmations of faith and services and so little humanity! Didn't that also have something to do with him?

Later I thought that Jesus must also have experienced a development. In the end, shortly before his death, he didn't say another word about faith but only used the solidarity with his "spiritual brothers" as a measure.

Once, the house mother brought those who were allowed to get up yarn for knitting. It was the only time during the eleven weeks I was on this ward that we were allowed to occupy ourselves. Like possessed ones we sat bent over our white cotton ankle socks with pink borders after the long, torturous period of doing nothing. Quiet descended on the "restless ward." Then the yarn ran out, the socks were delivered, and we became loud again. There were no kinds of games here. And our relatives who could so easily have sent us something with which to stay busy, apparently had no idea that we were simply being stored here.

When I was finally allowed to get up and even go out to the ward garden with the high wall, I was still uncertain about whether transformations were possible. Nurse Y. had given me a coffee table book with pictures to look at, and there was a painting of a woman who kneels before Jesus with raised arms, and branches sprouted from her fingers. "Noli me tangere!" it said underneath—apparently the woman was scared that Jesus could turn her into a tree by touching her. Better not to step on the grass, I told myself. Who knows who has been turned into grass in this eerie house.

How did I get to the fingers from which branches were sprouting? I asked myself later and later had an art library show me an art book about Fritz von Uhde,[8] because it could only have been his painting "Noli me tangere." The branches are sparse little trees at the center of the images, which start exactly above the splayed-out fingers of the kneeling woman's raised hands. It is about Mary Magdalene's encounter with the resurrected Jesus, and she doesn't seek to be touched by him, as I make out from her pleading raised hands, but rather he doesn't want to be touched by her.

It eventually dawned on me that the house was not capable of transformations. Now I felt confident enough to step on the little lawn on hot days and lie down under the round shade of the young linden tree. If I rolled myself into a little ball, I fit under it perfectly.

Once when I was walking around the lawn area, I saw the chief physician with a big, strong man—probably a colleague—standing on the ramp above; he seemed to be showing him the ward garden. The stranger looked at me steadfastly. I stopped and looked at him as steadfastly as he was looking at me. He didn't look uninteresting. But how unworthy, I thought, to observe us like animals in the zoo instead of talking to us! And even as I looked at both of them just as silently as they looked at me, I remained the prisoner and they remained the free ones. They could look down from the ramp into the partly walled and partly fenced-in zoo exhibit.

In the meantime, I knew we were being kept here because we were "mentally ill." And I had sworn to myself that I'd rather stay mentally ill than ever take part in having the "mental health" being demonstrated here; it seemed to me not worth aspiring to. Even if Nurse Y. sometimes took me into her arms, I did not trust the

8 Fritz von Uhde is a German painter who often painted religious subjects.

peace because she was only nice to us when we lay in our beds still and obediently.

On the last day of June, Nurse Y. told me my mother was there. A visitor for the first time—finally someone from home had come! Nurse Y. pushed me into the little visiting room that belonged to the ward. There, however, I did not find my mother. Two unknown men sat there bent over files.

Why had I gone into the moor, they wanted to know. For the first time someone was asking about the reason for my actions! But I couldn't talk about it to these completely unknown men. Evasively, I said that I had found it quite nice. I only had one thought in my mind, to get to my mother as soon as possible. I had no idea these two unknown men represented a "genetic health jury"[9] and that this was about my sterilization.

Why had I gone to the airport on our island, they asked further. Or: what was it I wanted at the airport. I don't know any longer what I answered. I was still too confused. How could all of that be in the files? Only the men at the airport I asked whether Molt and his wife had arrived yet knew anything about it. Those men probably told my parents.

Relatives have no idea that their statements are included in the patient report and can then be used against the patient. I don't remember what else these men asked. I was already sitting on the edge of my seat. That that meeting was supposed to be a trial! I hadn't been informed what this conversation was even about and had no possibility to defend myself. It was pure farce.

When I then told Mother about the conditions on the "restless ward" and about the "calming techniques," she did not think it sounded implausible. "You also told

9 Buck is referring to agents of the Nazi Hereditary, or Genetic, Health Courts who determined outcomes for diagnosed or otherwise suspect "sick" persons such as Buck.

Nurse Y. that she had placed a witch's lamp on your bed." That was true, I had said that. I imagined that the red-hot glowing spot on the bedcover, a result of her touch, had spread so fast it could have only been something as unreal as a witch's lamp. I didn't know anything yet about the symbolic meaning of hallucinations, after all. And for that reason, I was now thought untrustworthy, so Mother considered everything I told her about the institution to be imagined or made up! But in psychiatric textbooks she could have read that the duration baths and the "wet wraps" really existed!

I saw by her reaction that it made no sense to talk about my experiences on this ward. That was difficult for me because these experiences were the most oppressive ones of my life, much worse than it would be later, in 1944, to be stuck in the debris following a bomb attack.[10] An enemy bomb threatens one's life and elicits fear, but it doesn't discriminate. In the institution, on the contrary, we were robbed of our dignity; we were reduced to being objects to be kept and observed. We were objects to whom it was not worth talking, and who were not worthy of occupation or else considered incapable of being occupied. And to be unable to talk to anyone about it was the same as total inner isolation.

Mother told me Molt had written after I was admitted to Bethel, and how sorry he was to have been partially responsible for my becoming ill. She'd reassured him that this was not the case. I agreed with her. Feelings of guilt wouldn't have helped him or me. And I also couldn't believe that the development triggered in me was only sick or without value. As much as Bethel tried to fight my

10 The eight-day bombing of Hamburg in July of 1943, which Buck lived through, created a firestorm that killed between thirty-four thousand and forty-three thousand, making it more destructive than the firebombing of Dresden. It was known by the Allies as Operation Gomorrah.

experiences as the expression of "mental illness"—for me they remained something very essential.

4

The Procedure

After Mother's visit, I was moved to the adjacent "quiet ward." That too was a locked ward. It was older and darker but had a bigger garden surrounded by a high cinderblock wall, and in front of the ground floor dayroom there was a flowerbed. There had been no flowers in the smaller garden of the "restless ward," instead just bushes on a bed to the side. We'd only been able to look at the round rose bed through a high chain-link fence.

With the assistant (female) doctor I stood in front of the blue cornflowers being circled by buzzing bees. "Do you still remember that you said you were the bride of Christ?" she asked. How could I have forgotten, how could I ever forget the attack on that laundry morning! If she'd asked what was happening before that morning, I could have told her about my previous weeklong impatient attempts, and maybe she'd have understood what the identification with the symbolism of the bride meant.

Many years later, I asked why she and the other doctors and the nurses didn't talk to us. She just said: "The patients don't like it." We really don't like questions which from the start feel as if they are trying to devalue and make no attempt at understanding. But if the young doctor had said back then: such ideas break out of the usually unconscious state; let us try to figure out what it means to you to be the bride of Christ, then I would surely have been thankful. C.G. Jung would have done it similarly with his patients. When we afflicted feel understanding and that we are being taken seriously, that the sense of our experiences is not devalued right away, we certainly don't show the kind of reserve we're said to demonstrate. Later conversations with other patients, in which we spoke freely and openly about our experiences in psychosis, showed me this.

During her visit, Mother purchased two doilies to embroider. Now I at least had some handiwork. I liked to walk along the lawn under the old trees in the garden with my eyes closed and try to recognize them based on the sound of their leaves. The dark rustling of the great, gentle chestnut leaves shook out from the lighter sound of the other trees with their narrower and smaller leaves.

After a week I was moved again and now, for the first time, I came into a ward where I felt a little trust. It was completely different from the other two. The atmosphere in the hall with about ten beds, and the three smaller rooms, was caring. On the nightstands there were flower vases and during the day the beds were covered with decorative blankets which a former patient had crocheted with intricate patterns. In front of the hall there was a pavilion whose door to the little ward garden stood open, and this ward garden was only separated from the main garden by a low fence with an open gate. So, we also had free access to the beautifully planted large garden close by an ascending slope, with its pergola overgrown with roses. My favorite thing to do was to sit hidden under the low-hanging branches of a hanging, or "grief," beech.

The ward nurse M., who was about fifty, had an aura of goodness about her and sometimes even demonstrated a sense of humor. The second, still young nurse was also friendly. The depressed ones lay in this ward; compared to the schizophrenics they only seemed to be unhappy. Nurse M. tried to comfort them and calm them. Here they didn't use duration baths and wet applications, or cold-water showers on the head and sedative injections.

The other patients in this ward are not as present in my mind's eye as those from the "restless ward." Across from me was Miss von B., a woman of about forty, who had slit her wrists at home; the scars on them were still new. She still sat in bed, desperate; later she got up and calmed down. The gray-haired Miss H. seemed even more unhappy. I never saw this woman laugh the way Miss von B. did, at least once in a while. Driven by an inner restlessness, she constantly whispered words of self-accusation. An older Baltic woman brought a little bit of normalcy to the ward atmosphere due to her pleasant, broad tone of voice. She usually sat on the sofa of the little day room — the "restless ward" had only had wooden benches. The old lady sat bent over her artistic crochet work in one of the adjacent two bedrooms next to the hall. But for me, the most moving figure was a girl whose age I couldn't make out, who had a quiet and reserved grace. She came from a farm and wasn't here for the first time. We never spoke out loud with one another.

Here I experienced for the first time that the patients of this institution were not just fought against. The depressed also had consultations with the doctor; they received help. When three of us complained about the bad treatment in the "restless ward" to the house mother, she did not want to believe us. She clearly didn't want to recognize that the "calming measures" and the refusal to talk and keep us occupied could be considered abuse, because they were definitely doctors' orders. The intermittent beatings with the iron door handle attached to a leather belt were only noticed later, due to Little Marie G.'s injuries, and without such visible results no one usually believes patient complaints.

Now a very active correspondence with my parents and my siblings began. In July alone I received sixteen letters.

On July 12 my mother wrote:

> Now you know that you were ill. We kept you at home for as long as was possible. But then we had to accept that you, in order to get healthy again, had to receive appropriate care and then we looked for the best we could find among what we knew. And now we beg of you with all our hearts: don't lose your patience and don't lock yourself against the great love that you are surrounded by and which you feel. You can really depend on it: You won't stay in Bethel a day longer than you have to .... You write that you are completely healthy and physically you are. And because you don't have any pain and don't feel weak you don't understand that you are still being kept. The world of your thoughts was sick. And now we've repeatedly been told: in such situations don't release them too early so there are no relapses. And if you are now going to become impatient and start to get mad at your surroundings then you are holding up your recovery. You must find some peace inside around this topic and can't lose your faith. Doctors and nurses can help much better when the sick are willing to be helped.

Mother was right: this ward was caring. I felt the love. But the experiences in the "restless ward" couldn't be erased because of it. They were deeply imprinted; that's how people who can't defend themselves are treated.

On August 7, Mother wrote:

> Yes, patience. Youth doesn't like it and they quickly see it as weakness and lack of personality, and it is in fact in many cases strong collected power and you must now learn it at such a young age already. We feel it with you and know that your life isn't easy right now and understand if it sometimes appears gray to you and you long for the time in which you had a heightened sense of life. But darling, we want to trust that because of the heaviness something better will happen. Recently,

> a woman wrote to me who went through a lot of darkness especially spiritually: "I owe my best to the heaviest"....

And a week later:

> What sorts of accusations are you making toward us? Maybe it would be good if you were to talk about it. We would so very much like to help you. If I wrote to you of a good friend who owes the best in her life to the hardest, then I, of course, did not mean for you to see it that way already. That is utterly impossible. But it is an experience that innumerable people have over the course of their lives. And it is not as if those who seem to have the good and easy life seen from the outside, have the richest lives.

I couldn't understand at all that my mother saw my walk into the mudflats as a "darkness in the spiritual realm." Even in her card that she'd sent me off with to the mainland hospital ("And though I wandered in the dark valley..."), she had expressed that idea. She might have thought my walk was a suicide attempt. I thought that was unlikely because I'd told her about both the stars that rose in the sky, as if they were a miracle. After a suicide attempt, I would certainly not have asked right away for a piece of cake. No, the heaviness, and torturous thing, for me was not what I experienced internally but how I was treated because of it.

I was moved to a little single bedroom in the open ward but did not have permission to leave yet. On August 22, Father wrote:

> What happened has been hard for you, you sweetheart. But there is nothing you have to be embarrassed about. Only we must strive to get you in surroundings in which you don't think people are looking at you be-

> cause of it; instead one where you can internally develop freely in a state of healthy harmlessness. That is why I already took some steps in June.

He meant: for a transfer to a new rectorate.

My older sister wrote:

> That you now are in such a nice situation makes me very happy. I was especially happy to hear that you are interested in children again.... We were very sorry that you were sick. But hopefully you won't feel embarrassed about it around us. Of course we are sorry that we are moving. On the other hand, the parental home isn't actually our residence anymore.

One evening—it was September 17—the friendly ward nurse M. shaved my pubic hair after my bath. Why? I wanted to know. "For a necessary little procedure." It was obvious that she didn't want to provide a more detailed explanation and I didn't ask any further. I had no idea about a sterilization. That is why I hadn't had any doubts when Nurse Y. referred to my co-patient's scars as "appendix scars"; many, after all, had their appendices operated on. And I never would have thought it possible such a serious procedure could be done without first talking about it to the concerned party.

At home, it had been understood that I was informed of everything that concerned me. When my parents took me to the mainland hospital and then had me brought to Bethel without telling me where I was going, that understanding had changed for the first time, and I'd experienced that as a breach of trust. Here, however, in the institution, I clearly had no right to information about anything. One could do with me as one wished without losing a word over it.

Early in the morning, Nurse M. took me to the Gilead hospital. I felt no fear at all as I stood along in the antechamber of the operating room in my white cotton socks and short shirt. For the first time in more than five months I was able to open a window all the way, and I felt such happiness about this wide open window on a bright morning with the sun rising. I still had no idea what they planned to do with me.

Nurse M. entered and was visibly startled to see me standing at an open window. The thought of jumping out of it had never crossed my mind. She quickly closed the window and I got on the gurney that was rolled into the antechamber. The anesthesiology nurse — I still see her face — injected my arm and I sank into the unconsciousness I was already so familiar with, though it was faster than I was used to. This injection worked much faster than the ones that Nurse Y. jabbed into my thigh, once with such force that the discoloration of the skin can still be seen today.

I woke up out of anesthesia in the little four-bedroom area in the ward for the depressed. Now as well, nobody informed me what kind of procedure had been performed.

On September 23, a few days after the operation my mother wrote:

> My dear beloved child, we received news from Nurse R. and now know that you had the operation and are doing well. We didn't know that it had already been done or we would of course have already written. Of course you know that our thoughts are with you very, very much. How grateful and happy it made us that you live life so courageously; I have to tell you that today. That is what has comforted us the most these last months that we saw you were happy and believe that God's father hand is leading you even if the path seems dark. Almost twenty-six years ago we chose the following as our wedding quote: My thoughts are not your thoughts and my path is not your path. And now comes the "rather" that transforms the dark into the

> light: Rather, by the same measure that the sky is higher than the earth, my paths are higher than your paths and my thoughts than your thoughts. My Sophiechild, it is bitterly difficult for us that you must experience this at such a young age. The new state demands some things which are a great sacrifice for the individual. Here we are simply dictated to comply: everyone is subject to the authorities that be. But now God says something about the human demand: those who love God should be served best by all things. It will be of utmost importance to us parents to help you so that your life turns out well. You know, I have thought on occasion how much the German people need women who are not biological mothers and yet still have a motherly heart. I have often seen how much more love unmarried women have for children. With mothers, love gets worn out for their own children so fast. In that area there are so many tasks — and now we want to be happy that this mountain has been overcome. It first had to be done, of course, before one could talk about plans for the future.

Another patient, a deaconess who had been living here a long time following a car accident, explained to me that the operation was a sterilization. She had brought flower garlands she made herself to my sickbed. Without her I would probably not have found out anything in this house.

I was in despair. I had my hair cut, because I at least wanted to watch my hair grow if everything else in my development was to stop. I didn't feel like a real woman anymore. Made infertile because of mental inferiority! Not being able to have children! Not being able to marry! Not being able to become a kindergarten teacher! Not being able to learn or work in any kind of social profession! What was left for me to do?

Everything had been in vain. My resistance to the inhumane "reason" of the "restless ward" that they tried to convert us to — in vain. My refusal against everything with which they tried to bow our wills and confuse us ever more deeply — in vain. Nurse M. had played down the operation as a "necessary little procedure." It wasn't a "little procedure," it was a terribly big infringement on my whole future life. They overpowered me when they shoved me into that little visitation room, not telling me the two strange men were going to make a ruling about my sterilization.

"Can be sterilized through surgical procedure," it said in the sterilization law of July 25, 1933. Thus, doctors were given space to judge.

Mother had told the chief physician that my psychosis probably had emotional reasons; that's what she later told me. The chief physician had responded that the psychosis would have come out regardless, even without any kind of emotional shock. Mother had absolute faith in doctors. How should she have known that doctors didn't talk to the psychotics and so had no idea what was going on inside of them and why they had turned psychotic?

Soon after the operation, Mother visited me and later wrote:

> God allowed you to get sick. He sent us and you great pain by doing that. I believe you always think that you are the one who worries us. That is a very wrong thought. No, this suffering comes from God and he will have known that we needed hard times. And now we'll simply try to stay quiet and will try to learn from it what we are supposed to learn, you and us.... If we try to accept it as something God has sent, and when we have seriously asked for the sin to be taken from us and forgiven (for, of course, one sees much more clearly what one has done wrong), then surely a great blessing will come from all of this heaviness.

Ten days later she wrote:

> It is a great joy to see that you are fighting off the sad thoughts. Fighting is the main thing and if it doesn't work right away then we will accept it from God's hand. Perhaps he wants to show us our complete helplessness so that we turn to him completely and expect everything of him.... If you are not able to get over the situation with the X-ray then tell the house mother and ask her whether it's possible that you experienced something like that.

And then again:

> We ask from our hearts with you and for you that you are able to let go of the thoughts of the past. That actually is the illness, that you cannot see things properly, some things, in many things you are just like you used to be, but there are still some remnants that have stayed that simply must go away. And the sooner you can shake it off, the sooner you can go back to ward 1 and then we can also begin to plan for the future again. Maybe it would be helpful if when the sad thoughts come, you sing or try to learn a song? I am now learning "O come, you spirit of truth." It is by Spitta, whom Grandmother loved especially....

When I recently found my parents' letters in my old doll case, I was moved by their love and their piety. Back then, apparently, doubt about whether the "spirit of truth" could be instilled by learning a chorale prevailed. What if the fire I experienced under my cover, and whose results still give me a hard time, and the disappeared mudflats' water weren't also truths I couldn't just "shake off?" Did *they* see things the right way? They didn't even know what I had experienced and what the meaning of these experiences was for me. They simply believed the assertions of the chief physician that my psychosis had nothing to do with previously experienced emotional shock and would have broken out regardless. They would just as definitely have accepted a psychotherapist's opinion, who would have understood my psychosis just the way I experienced it. And then we could have talked about the reasons and connections to attain real understanding, instead of suppressing them, and having them be a hindrance to healing in the short term.

And Mother couldn't know how difficult it was for me to accept the sterilization from God's hand. I had, in fact, thought I was following his lead. She knew nothing about the reasons for my psychosis. So now everything was supposed to have been a mistake, just a mental illness! I had to admit that the "terrible war" I had expected in the immediate future would not break out. And so the "bride of Christ" had also only been a delusion, although the identification with the symbol made it possible to realize I had to develop my own personality and my gut told me that I had understood this correctly. And it was also not normal that I followed the morning star into the mudflats; in a normal state I would not have felt any kind of impulse to do so. Why did you let me go astray? I argued. You knew I would believe the inner voice as your voice!

But a quiet doubt remained: the mudflats water that disappeared. Armgard's father, Pastor Th., a mudflats expert, had made a sketch and wrote about it like this:

> About one and a half to two kilometers south of the island the first eddy extends, and it is used by little ships during high tide and to cross between the island and mainland in the west–east direction. Hence this eddy is marked by poles whose bushy tips still stick out during high tide. At the highest (i.e., shallowest) spot where the mudflats wanderer can walk onto mainland, there is a buoy at the north shore of the eddy. This is also where the cable from the mainland crosses the

> eddy. The buoy serves as a warning for ships not to anchor here because a dragging anchor could damage the cable or completely rip it out.

The north shore where the buoy lay was the island side. How could I have reached the eddy crawling, after I had shortly before followed the morning star in a southerly direction by swimming through it? Even the shallowest spot was never dry. I couldn't find an obvious answer for the disappearance of the water. If the drying up was only about saving me from a life-threatening situation when I sank in the mud, then just a little bit more strength should have been enough for me to swim back. So why had the water disappeared? And why did the pastors still teach stories like the one of Abraham's test of obedience if God's guidance couldn't be experienced in a way that defied all reason? Why did they still teach Jesus's miracles if such miracles were only allowed to exist in the distant past? If He did not have the strength today, then his words about a faith that could move mountains was just an old saying.

But even if it were true that I'd followed God's guidance, I would still have been branded as an "inferior, mentally ill woman" and would have had to live with this mark at least sixty years, judging by our family's longevity. That is an unimaginably long time for a nineteen-year-old. But my quiet doubt of the validity of the psychiatric evaluation seemed to help me more than I could see in my desperation back then. It probably was what saved me from the "personality disintegration" that schizophrenics supposedly can't avoid suffering, as can be read in the encyclopedia. This "disintegration" is in fact a falling apart with oneself. It happens through the psychiatric invalidation of the psychosis experiences as "meaningless" and "mentally ill" that self-confidence is destroyed — if we do believe this evaluation. And who could dodge this evaluation if they have not had the experiences which egg on doubt?

The doctors noticed my desperation and moved me from the open to the closed ward for the depressed, so back to Nurse M. That's where I stayed until I was discharged. Although my depression was only natural and understandable following the operation, they still did not talk to me, and I can only explain their silence by thinking they had ordered the sterilization and subsequently were trying to avoid a conversation.

An acting student was brought in by her mother. She seemed completely vacuous. Nurse M. led her through the hall into one of the adjacent little rooms, brought her to her bed, and put up a screen in front of the bed to spare her having to see all the depressed women. Envy filled me on account of this show of care. What would have happened if Mother had accompanied me here? If my parents had not left me in the dark mainland hospital over Easter, with the room with bars and the caretakers' teasing? If I had arrived here just as trustingly as I left home? Perhaps I would have been put into this friendly ward right away, and I wouldn't have had to endure all of the ridiculous calming measures, which didn't exist here. I wouldn't have been greeted with a little glass of paraldehyde and nobody would have wished me a "good night on my wedding night." All these terrible fears wouldn't have had to surface, that the "city of charity" was a lie and that everything we had learned perhaps was not right. Would I have then still been sterilized?

And didn't it seem obvious that patients who were delivered at the institution without being accompanied by family members were treated with less care than those whose families showed interest, so their children couldn't be treated as if they had no worth? Later the acting student told me that the chief physician had spoken with her and told her he knew about depressions; they were worse than having one's belly cut open. With the depressed on this ward there were medical consults with doctors.

I was invited to Mother's friend, who was married to a Bethel theologian, for Christmas. She was very nice to me, but I remained depressed because my situation seemed to me hopeless.

On this ward a book found its way into my hands. In the book a woman nearly froze to death in a winter forest — either due to a mishap or because she was looking for death. The thought of suicide had never entered my mind till then, although I saw the scars on Miss von B.'s wrists daily; her failed attempt could only have a discouraging effect. After I finished this book, I felt the ground under my feet again. So, there was a way to end this seemingly meaningless life of an inferior mentally ill person, and it was possible to end life in such a way that it looked like an accident. Because an unambiguous suicide would have been too great a sorrow for my parents and something I didn't want to do to them. When instead of sixty years, which seemed like an infinity, I only looked one or two or five years ahead, my desperation already seemed to lift a little. Because the hopelessness lay in the unpredictability of the time span that lay ahead of me. With the thought of suicide, I could predict an end. Without a goal people cannot live; now I had a goal again after my life goal had been taken away from me. I was able to plan again even if it was the freedom of suicide.

In one year, I decided. Or in two years. I could fill that much time even with this heavy burden of being marked as "inferior." My strength, bound by desperation, could flow toward life again. Without this self-imposed deadline of first one and later a number of years, I would not have had the strength to keep living; the thought of an infinitely long period of time that lay before me and that I would have had to get through, one with the sacrifice of so much that belongs to a real life, would have paralyzed me. Many who were forcibly sterilized are said to have ended their lives.

After a year, the situation already looked a little different for me, although I was still deeply insecure. I set myself a new deadline, but already not with the same decisiveness, that I would really end this. A few times I extended the deadlines until, very much later, I didn't need them anymore.

But I have repeatedly asked myself why Bethel didn't show more care and responsibility toward the affected when delivering such a measure deeply impacting on a life's fate, not to at least have a conversation with us before the sterilization order was applied. Every offender, even back then, had a right to defense; we, however, could not defend ourselves, couldn't present the emotional reasons for our psychoses to the genetic health court because we weren't even informed what this process was all about. That silence was even illegal according to the sterilization law of July 25, 1933, because this law at least acknowledged the right of the person in question to be informed beforehand. In §2.2 it rules: "The application is to include a certificate from a physician who has been approved by the German Reich, which attests that the person to be sterilized has been instructed about the nature and the effects of the sterilization." This information requirement is not lifted in any paragraph for the sterilization applications of the institution director.

How much easier would it have been for us to bear the sterilization if we had been informed that doctors and nurses were working on our behalf but could not save us from the operation!

I found a partial answer to all these questions in 1964 in the book *Protestant Documents about the Murder of the "Incurably Ill" under the National Socialist Rule for the Years*

1939-1945, published that same year.[1] In excerpts one can find quotes from the minutes of a meeting of the Central Committee for the Internal Mission's specialized conference for eugenics, which was held May 1931 in Treysa near Kassel; the full transcript was published by Bethel in 1983 in its "Readings on the Issues of 'Eugenics, Sterilization, Euthanasia.'" Among the twenty-three participants of the meeting were seven senior physicians as well as nine directors of Protestant institutions for epileptics, those deemed "idiots," and mentally ill. The meeting was about, among other things, "demands for the simplification and price reduction of the care measures for the inferior and antisocial." The transcript reads as following about the results:

> The structural changes within our population composition and the quantitative as well as qualitative change of population increase, which shows especially in the shrinking of average family size among the groups of the genetically and socially able and productive, make... a *eugenic reorientation of our public and free social services* urgently needed. Instead of undiscriminating socialized care, there must be *differentiated care.* Significant expenses should only be paid for such groups requiring care who will likely regain their full productivity. But for all others, socialized care measures should be limited to what is fit for human care and holding. Those who carry genetic traits that cause social inferiority and require care should under all circumstances be barred from procreation....
>
> God gave humans soul and body, he gave them the responsibility for both — not, however, the right, to

1 Evangelische Kirche in Deutschland, *Evangelische Dokumente zur Ermordung der „unheilbar Kranken" unter der nationalsozialistischen Herrschaft in den Jahren 1939–1945*, ed. Hans Christoph von Hase (Stuttgart: Evangelisches Verlagswerk, 1964).

> freely vacillate.... When these God-given functions lead to evil or destruction of his kingdom in one or the other link of the community, then not just a right, but a moral responsibility exists for sterilization as an act of neighborly love. It is our responsibility not just for the generation that has come into existence but for the coming one.... In order to counteract abuses in this area, it appears most desirable to this conference that the sterilization of the individual in question happen without an appeal and not be considered personal injury in a criminal sense, as long as it occurred because of eugenic social indications and was carried out according to the rules of the medical arts.[2]

These demands were made two years before Hitler's power grab.

Why did the theological institution directors and the leading physicians of Protestant institutions see a role for themselves in population politics? They were supposed to be responsible for helping their patients. They called on Christian standards to replace them with political viewpoints on population. The "neighborly love" with which they argued the "moral obligation" for sterilization certainly did not pertain to the affected but rather to the institution directors and doctors.

Here, patients were being called "inferior and antisocial elements." The nine institution directors and seven lead physicians didn't seem to ask themselves how they valued human beings who were only granted "what is fit for humane care and holding"—as if simply holding could ever be humane. They could hardly do anything worse than simply holding their patients. No incarcerated person was subjected to this yearlong monotony

2 Arbeitskreis "Geschichte Bethels," ed., *Lese-Texte zur Problemkreis "Eugenik, Sterilisation, Euthanasie"* (Bethel bei Bielefeld: Verlagshandlung der Anstalt Bethel, 1983), 69–72.

and lack of occupation. With the resulting slow decline, a lethal injection could ultimately even be a relief.

On the "restless ward" the nurses were focused primarily on preventing suicides, and it seems that is necessary where patients are only held and thus cannot see meaning in their lives anymore. But it's the institution's fault and not the patient's. A person who not only has lost their freedom but every possibility to occupy themselves loses their self-confidence. The care personnel then considers them incapable and unworthy of their respect because they appear to be so apathetic. But it is the other way around: they become apathetic because they are treated as incapable and without respect. And with all of that, the calming measures for those held without an occupation were more costly than occupation would have been, as it was introduced in 1923 for all patients in the nearby Gütersloh institution.

When in the fall of 1939 the patient murders of the "euthanasia" set in, productivity was a deciding factor for death or survival. But held patients had no way of being productive. At least Bethel didn't fill out the forms for the euthanasia action.[3] The result of this refusal was, as the assistant doctor wrote in a letter to the editor in *Spiegel* (May 17, 1961),

> the appearance of an SS commission in Bethel, to which among others, the professors Kihn from Jena and Carl Schneider from Heidelberg belonged. We were forced to present our ill patients while the SS doctors filled out the forms, while we desperately tried to present the ill patients as being social and productive.[4]

3 Questionnaires addressing category of illness and ability to work were filled out by doctors of their own patients, then processed for a life-or-death decision at T4 headquarters in Berlin. These decisions were rendered with plus or minus signs on the form.

4 Letter from Dr. Med. Gertrud Runge in the section "Briefe," *Spiegel*, May 16, 1961, https://www.spiegel.de/politik/sterbehilfe-a-

How much easier would it have been if the patients had in fact had real opportunities to occupy themselves! And aside from the two older women who were close to dying and apathetic Little Marie, in 1936 everyone in Bethel would have been glad to have something to do. But the patients' needs didn't count. Nobody wondered whether it was caring or social to just treat us like objects of observation and storing, not to deem us worth talking to, but to submit sterilization order forms for, or rather, against us. They only saw *their* reality: the psychiatric dogma of meaningless symptoms of a physical illness due to a genetic burden.

They did not see our reality at all: our experience in psychosis, the history that led to it, and the meaning it had for us. They knew nothing of this and didn't want to know anything of this because to do so would have required them engaging in conversations open to understanding. We patients were much more "community-oriented" (which back then was a criterion for "euthanasia") among ourselves.

Pastor Fritz von Bodelschwingh[5] also supported the resolutions of Treysa.[6] In the Bodelschwingh biography by Wilhelm Brandt it says he was "very soon known and admired ... in all the most important subcommittees of the Central Committee for Internal Mission, such that his advice set the tone in many personnel and procedural decisions."[7] One can hardly assume that he wasn't heard regarding such significant decisions even if he did not participate in the conference.

4b52ac67-0002-0001-0000-000043364022. Buck erroneously dates the issue to May 17.

5 This pastor was the nephew and namesake of the Pastor von Bodelschwingh who ran Bethel during Buck's imprisonment there.

6 The Treysa Conference in 1945 created a new, united Evangelical Church, but failed to acknowledge complicity in Nazi crimes.

7 Wilhelm Brandt, *Friedrich von Bodelschwingh, 1877–1946* (Bethel bei Bielefeld: Verlagshandlung der Anstalt Bethel, 1949), 87.

In the *Zeit* from April 18, 1986, Ernst Klee reported:

> In 1945, Pastor v. Bodelschwingh was of the opinion that the law[8] was a help, as there had been a need, particularly for regulations for idiots. He refused to endorse compensation because reparation claims would have brought up new grief around the sterilized: "Were one to even give the sterilized the right to claim reparations," the minutes of the reparations committee of the parliament states, "then it would just bring anxiety and new, heavy suffering to the individuals who don't have a bigger understanding of these things."[9]

That reparations would cause "new, heavy suffering" I find a strange justification. Because Bethel's pastors and doctors didn't mention or care about the suffering we experienced back then, which was not just an assumed state but a very real one. Anyone who listened to those affected would know reparations for the lifelong burden of forcible sterilization would have decisively made it easier, because it would have lifted the sentence of "inferiority." It would, of course, have been more difficult for the directors and doctors of the institutions of the Internal Mission if what had been described as "neighborly love" was declared wrong.

Today, Bethel tries "to be aware of its own past in order to simultaneously gain insights for a path into the future,"[10] as Pastor Johannes Busch, the current

8 Nazi Hereditary Disease Law.

9 Ernst Klee, "Geldverschwendung an Schwachsinnige und Säufer," *Die Zeit* 18 (1986), https://www.zeit.de/1986/18/geldverschwendung-an-schwachsinnige-und-saeufer/komplettansicht.

10 Johannes Busch, "Vorwort," in Arbeitskreis "Geschichte Bethels," ed., *Lese-Texte zur Problemkreis "Eugenik, Sterilisation, Euthanasie."* The editor has attempted to trace back all of Buck's citations to their original German sources. As many of them are no longer easily accessible, some page numbers remain missing.

director of Bethel, wrote in 1983 in the foreword to the "Readings Around the Issues of 'Eugenics, Sterilization, Euthanasia.'" But those insights include the experiences we affected had, and the lifelong consequences that the forcible sterilization had and still has. Perhaps they wouldn't have been completely meaningless if they could contribute to a "path into the future."

I experienced my four later breaks clearly due to being branded as an "inferior mentally ill woman"; I needed something to balance out this human devaluation. That is why they developed more unavoidably than my first break. I experienced the first one as an important developmental phase for myself in which I still had opportunities to make decisions freely. After Molt left, everything could have pulled itself together again, and I knew that I had to make a decision. But I had the feeling that the collapse made sense and would cause something new, while the re-establishment of the old state would have been a retreat.

When I was unable to find a relationship with Jesus, in spite of my best efforts, and in the fifth week experienced the at-first still quiet epiphanies and internal impulses, I decided consciously to give up my will, and follow this inner voice which represented God's guidance for me. After the two stars rose, I paid careful attention to the internal impulse to head out, which allowed me to follow the shining path of the morning star on the wet mudflats. On heading out, I experienced this walk to the mudflats as the foreshadowing of a development I had to catch up with. After the first walk to the sea, the music stopped in exactly the same moment that my life threatened to continue in the straight ditch of entrenched habits. Now the new path was leading me to rebirth from the mud and I experienced the sun rise, the sun which during my first sea walk, and in the music I heard, had stayed hidden.

But it was only through a change from my normal way of being that this symbol could gain this overwhelming meaning. And that I could experience the two rising stars as a miracle, without thinking they might possibly always appear this way. This changed experience of the world became clearer to me in my later breaks. During my fourth or fifth break, I called them "central experiences," because all areas of human life, which in "normal" world experience are split up without a relationship to one another, I experienced as meaningfully connected and unified, as in a hand-held fan whose segments all arise from a common center.

5

Liberation during the Break

The doctors had no idea what had given me new drive, and they could hardly have had an idea because they didn't talk to me. The beginning or the middle of January 1937, they discharged me. Confused but undamaged in spirit, I'd been taken away from home three-quarters of a year ago. Deeply bewildered, with the suicide plan as my only perspective for the future, I left Bethel. My mother picked me up. We rode to my grandmother and aunt's. I was not to return to the island.

What was now to become of me? There was only one career I was allowed to pursue and perform; all other paths were closed to me. I longed to go into vocational training as quickly as possible. Only this way would I have the freedom to commit suicide, which gave me the power to live.

My grandmother lived in a little place along the Rhine. My mother stayed till the middle of April; she probably didn't want to transfer the responsibility for me to my grandmother and my aunt. I had been diagnosed as an "especially serious case of schizophrenia." I learned that later from Father, who also told me the chief physician had been especially interested in my "case." However, the doctor didn't show this interest, as he had not sought a conversation with me a single time.

At the movies, I saw a film about pottery-making in the previews. That seemed to be work cut out for me. On my twentieth birthday, the pastor of the town drove my mother and me to Höhr-Grenzhausen in the Westerwald. We looked at two pottery workshops and the ceramics institute. The mountains of the Westerwald, the raw climate, frost and snow in the wintertime—that was exactly what I needed. I could go skiing in the winter, could get lost in the forest, fall asleep and freeze to death in my sleep, and nobody would recognize this death as a suicide.

When I saw the students' sculptures at the institute, I felt the desire to do that, too. I had never worked with clay; my only attempts at modeling consisted of working on a Punch head out of papier-mâché, and a gray fabric donkey filled with sawdust for a nativity. The prerequisite for being accepted into the school was a completed pottery apprenticeship or a one-year ceramics internship. I also wanted to learn to use the potter's wheel, but that was only done by the men in both workshops we visited. That is why we decided on a primitive farmer's pottery workshop close by the city in which I had grown up.

In these months of constantly being with my mother, it would have been so obvious to talk about my psychosis. And also about how deeply bewildered I was that these experiences so important for me were supposedly only symptoms of a mental illness and entirely meaningless. Mother recognized how desperately I needed to talk. But she couldn't talk to me about these things. Because the chief physician, after all, had told her my psychosis had nothing to do with previous spiritual shocks and would have broken out regardless, independent of anything, and although Mother apparently was initially convinced that my "illness" had spiritual reasons, she relied on the doctor's authority. And so she made an appointment for me with a psychiatric female doctor in Düsseldorf who was supposed to be Christian and especially nice. I drove to see her in April 1937.

I can still see the doctor in my mind's eye, how she sat across from me at her desk: a woman around fifty, slim, short-haired, with blue eyes, vital. To help me she would have had to know the history of my psychosis and its contents. In a single conversation that took about an hour I couldn't say anything to a stranger I was seeing for the first time. And she did not even ask about it. Certainly, she shared the opinion so common at the time that psychoses were "endogenous," in other words, caused only physically, and that there was no sense in listening to content. I can hardly remember a word of our conversation and only know that I hesitantly presented my deep bewilderment.

On May 4, 1937, I began my internship year in the farmer's pottery workshop. The almost eighty-year-old master still dug for his own clay. He taught me to knead and use the potter's wheel with the same method he'd learned as an apprentice: a thousand flowerpots made to measure. The firing still took place in the traditional way in a large, self-made kiln. Day and night we threw the peat sods we'd dug up nearby into the two long fire troughs.

During the first weeks, my older sister stayed with me in the village. We lived in the great room of an old farmhouse. But then she had to return to work and with that the good order in the room disappeared. I gained joy in making pottery and also started to sculpt, but that didn't change anything with regard to my deep self-doubt. "Everything has become dark inside of me," I wrote to Molt. "How am I to differentiate between what comes from God and what comes out of me?"

After more than a year, this was the first letter to him. Back then, my letter had been hopeful and long, this one was short and gloomy.

It was very unpleasant to me now that I'd written so comprehensively back then, sharing "so much about myself and my thoughts." It had just come out of me like that, I wrote to him, and I hadn't even thought about the fact that he would read it, because "I certainly didn't want to lecture you." For me this long letter had been an expression of my trust and now I was embarrassed to have possibly been a burden. Nonetheless, I still felt a strong connection to him and was convinced he would be able to help me out of the deep self-doubt. He more than anyone could tell me whether what I had experienced as God's guidance was really just the delusion of a mentally ill woman. I still couldn't believe that. The transformation along the path by the sea into music had been something so overpowering—how could something like that be unhealthy?

I wasn't even sure whether he might not have come after all, following my urgent call from the hospital that evening when we were already in bed; since we'd set off early in the morning, we may have missed one another. Just to be sure I included many stamps in my letter to make up the difference for the possible trip. I imagined how Molt's wife may have reacted to the telephone call. "Sophie Zerchin just called from A.," Molt might have said. "She was at the doctor's with her mother and demanded I come right away."—"And, what did you say?"—"Of course, that I wouldn't come." How was it to continue now? Maybe she had asked this question sooner than he did and changed his mind to come after all. "I am not quite sure," I wrote, "whether you didn't in fact come. But after you said that you wouldn't come, I couldn't ask for you in the hospital anymore but just waited for you to make a start again." A fantastical assumption: that he could have come without announcing himself! Behind it certainly was my wish that he didn't simply leave me to my fate after my visit with the doctor.

Molt sent the stamps back—they were different ones. That he first used my stamps up satisfied me. He hoped, he wrote, I wasn't mad if a letter from him was arriving now. But he felt the urge to answer me. He had not been in A. back then. One can only understand a letter if one imagines the writer as vividly as if he were personally standing in front of one. That's when I realized just how deeply I must have hurt his feelings when I wrote about the impression he first made on me. That he had appeared two-sided because he did not approve or devalue his inner nature was something he obviously had not understood and probably was incapable of understanding back then.

He did not address my central question at all: how one could recognize what was coming from God and not out of oneself. I cannot remember what else he wrote. I was much too depressed and clearly also disappointed that he did not see my affection for him; without this affection I couldn't have written to him that at first, he hadn't seemed very nice.

Mother wrote to me: "Whenever you are seeking advice about anything, you can now write to Ms. Dr. W. because she is such a likable person." Ms. Dr. W.—that was the doctor from Düsseldorf. But how was she supposed to be able to help me? She hadn't even asked about my experiences of psychosis, clearly only saw them as meaningless side effects of a physical illness.

Until the middle of October, I stayed with my old master; after that I learned to glaze and duplicate in molds in a factory until the end of April 1938. Sundays I sculpted. For Christmas I sent home a sculpture of fired clay. Mother wrote: "We continue to find joy in your Christmas present. I ask myself how you actually made it. Did it evolve in your imagination or did someone model for you? I really wish you could now start sculpting. That and using the potter's wheel seems to me the nicest part of your work."

At the end of February, my parents moved to the new rectorate. So, now I could visit them again because nobody knew me there, nobody knew of my illness. After finishing my internship year, I stayed with them through the end of May.

How much money would it take to have my own ceramics workshop? Father asked a ceramics master. We would have to calculate start-up capital of ten thousand Reichsmark for a clay preparation machine, potter's wheel, kiln, and other tools. We didn't have these ten thousand Reichsmark. As a sculptor, however, I only needed a modeling stand. But was I talented enough to be a sculptor? I had taken my first stab at sculpting in the farmhouse ceramic workshop; among other things, I'd modeled in clay one of the kid goats that ran after me through the hedge paths to the ceramics workshop. It was just coming out of the kiln when a gentleman from Leipzig arrived. "That sweet little calf!" He wanted to have it right away. For 2.5 RM he bought it still warm. That was a good omen for me. I had also made first portrait attempts. The prospect of being able to express myself in clay filled me with new hope.

A woman sculptor was to test my talent. After the first week of June, I traveled to her for a month. She lived in the same city Molt did and in which the friend with whom I'd run the children's playgroup was getting her training. The old gentleman in whose house she lived with a fellow student also had a room for me.

I could have simply asked for a conversation with Molt. But after all the misunderstandings in our relationship and the stress of my psychosis, that didn't seem possible anymore. I was still too deeply insecure. But I called his former singing teacher; Molt had recommended him in case we ever wanted to consider schooling my voice further. Somehow, I must have hoped the singing teacher could mediate between Molt and me. Nobody answered the telephone.

The sculptor left her basement studio with tools and material for a month. With a burning zeal I jumped in, sculpting in a larger format than I had tried before. One morning I was bicycling in the street in which a singer lived, very close by. Nobody opened the apartment door. When I went back out on the street a light, apparently brand-new car was parked in front of the door; a gentleman with a stiff hat was just locking it. That is the gentleman who was sitting next to Molt in the car, ran through my mind — back then on the ride to Bethel, at the crossing in Halle! But back then the car had been dark. Attentively and silently, we gazed at each other. Then I took my bicycle, propped against the front garden gate, and rode back to the studio.

Later I called him, and we agreed on a first singing lesson. Even though I had no money to pay for the lesson, I would just sell a sculpture; that didn't seem so hard to me after the first terracotta piece had been bought still warm. He offered me a barter deal: singing lessons for a sculpture. I thought it was a good proposition.

He suggested the song of the linden tree by the well in front of the gate; I sang it and he accompanied me at the grand piano. "You have a beautiful voice but it's small," he said. "How did you find me of all people?" — "Because of a song weekend." — "Who organized it?" — "Molt." — "Was a sister of yours there?" With his head lowered he sat over the keys and played quietly. It took me by surprise, and I stuttered: Yes, my sister had attended the second conference. Only Molt could have known that, because at the second singing conference only islanders had attended. None of them knew the singer. Why had Molt told him about me? And what else had he said? There I was going to an unknown singer in a new city, and he knew I was mentally ill. Because it was certain that Molt had also told him, I simply assumed that. Because otherwise the singer would have said more. I was already familiar with this silence. I was not spoken to, but spoken about, and as if it was just to say: "She now seems to make a very healthy impression."

Maybe Molt had only spoken about me because he felt guilty at the thought that he was part of the reason for my psychosis breaking out; the singer was his friend. But I didn't think about it this way back then. After having been devalued in my humanity the way I was in Bethel, and being marked with the stain of the mentally ill woman, I could hardly imagine not being spoken about in a devaluing or in a pitying way. Under normal circumstances I would probably have asked right back: "How do you know that?" But someone who is branded as "mentally ill" cannot be so unselfconscious anymore. To what extent would my question embarrass him? What else did he know about me? The opportunity for a mediator between Molt and me had been so close, but that opportunity was now over. His unuttered knowledge and my insecurity stopped a conversation from the start.

It wasn't till much later I realized it wasn't Molt who'd spoken about me. The singer arrived at the first singing lesson a little late; a student had opened the door for me. He'd probably told her I was coming and also stated my name. And maybe she said: "Sophie Zerchin — I know her. We went to the same school. I thought she was ill and was in Bethel. But that could also be one of her sisters." That the student must have known about my illness only dawned on me much later in 1936, when I found a pile of letters from friends and acquaintances of my parents. All expressed their sympathy regarding this stroke of fate that hit my parents due to my psychosis. Included was a letter from the father of this past pupil, who was a former colleague of my father's. An old friend of my mother's wrote about a cognitively impaired boy who lived in an asylum but could recite the Lord's Prayer without a mistake and very movingly, in order to console her. How had my mother presented me to this friend, whom I didn't know was still in contact with her? And why was she still saving this letter? Too bad you don't have a cognitively impaired daughter I told myself as I read the letters; you would have been able to give her so much support with your experiences!

Actually, the singer's behavior should have shown me that the talk going around about me was not devaluing. He was full of human warmth and showed real interest in my work. Nonetheless, my insecurity grew. What might Molt have said about me? During a singing break, the singer told me about a lady who'd written a long letter. In her letter she accurately inferred things about him just based on her observations of his appearance and hand movements while singing Christ in the St. Matthew's Passion. At that moment he was addressing the budding sculptor in me; but I still had a hunch that Molt might have told him I'd taken myself to be the "bride of Christ." And when he explained the resonance of the voice in the head and said that the top of the skull vibrated and sometimes even buzzed, and then added: "You know that already," I wondered whether Molt told him I'd thrown a sink at the male nurse's head and hit him with it — surely, the top of his skull had also buzzed.

What could Armgard's father, who had driven me from the mainland hospital to Bethel, have told him about me? Certainly, her father had been told in the hospital why I was sitting in the basement. He was the only one who could have told Molt about my admission to Bethel, so Molt could right away write to my parents and say how sorry he was to have contributed to my illness. Armgard's father had stayed in touch with Molt following the first singing weekend, visited him with his children, and even stayed with him. And what may Molt have passed along to the singer? As absurd as all these speculations may seem — from the complete isolation of a former institution patient with whom nobody dared to talk openly, they are understandable to me today. I can still reconstruct the feeling of uncertainty this supposedly harmless question about my sister triggered in me. At any rate, under these circumstances, it was only burdensome to live in the same town as Molt.

That week we did a half-hour of voice and breathing exercises. We stayed on the song of the linden tree. "I dreamt in its shadow one or the other sweet dream," it goes. "You must also imagine something during it!" the singer said. I could only think about the young linden tree in the little ward garden with the high wall, in whose shadow I'd lain curled up. Sweet dreams had not filled me during that time, but instead the threatening reality of a type of "reasoning" that fought against whatever it didn't agree with.

I felt so fulfilled when one of the singer's students passed her voice teacher exam and I was allowed to be her student. "She sang wonderfully," I stated in the next lesson. I wished I could produce such a strong and full, diaphragmatically well-supported tone. "I can now hold the note for fifty seconds without taking another breath," I said. The singer was surprised I was looking at the clock while doing it. As with first attempts to swim, instead of being held by the water, I was being held by the tone. But I should not force it, he said. My mother wrote: "But that was a little bit careless with the concert singer. You didn't know the man at all."

I worked intensely in the basement studio. I had sculpted a relief and two larger sculptures, "Mother and Child"—a topic that would occupy me for decades. One sculpture that I called "Pain" seemed to almost form itself. It was made of coarse-grained fireclay, a material that forces large and simple forms. It was the figure of a kneeling woman, rearing up in pain with her head bent backward and her fists propped up on her thighs; the straight arms were pressed against her body and, with her backside, created a closed block or a kind of trunk. Even I was moved by the strong expression of this figure; it was a little uncomfortable. Because it was my own pain that I had expressed involuntarily, but I had to hide this pain and now as I saw it so directly in front of me, I did not even want to take ownership. For the cause of this pain was a stain that I had to keep secret; nobody was supposed to notice anything. How could we dare to show our pain at having been devalued in the institution and to express our rage! That would have been an admission of being a mentally ill woman in an institution; it would only bring us humiliating pity and new devaluation and thus would increase our isolation.

When twenty-six years later, I for the first time tried to write down the account of my illness, I soon had to give up because the rage rose in me, the rage about the suffered devaluation and the help refused to me was just too great; I had not even been aware of the intensity of it until then. The suppression of our feelings as well as the necessity to separate our psychosis experience as something meaningless from ourselves seems to me the worst thing that the psychiatric ward does to us. In Bethel, after my sterilization, I couldn't let anyone see my desperation in order not to endanger being discharged. Because all strong emotions were considered sick and were fought as if they were resistance. Every emotion, regardless of how justified, was thus suppressed into the unconscious. Even today, psychiatric wards still fight the emotions of the patients with an arsenal of emotion-suppressing measures: anesthesia, prolonged sleep, emotion-reducing psychotropic drugs. And after we've been discharged, the stain we have as "mentally ill" forces us to be so assimilated and inconspicuous, as is supposed to be normal, that we are actually for the most part denying our real feelings.

Probably it's exactly the suppressing of emotions that's a decisive prerequisite for the development of psychoses; at least the psychosis tends that way. For me it was the suppressed feeling of childhood disadvantage that needed to be counteracted. The devaluation as a "mentally ill" woman strengthened the emotional tension and thus makes new breaks a necessity. The psychiatric ward should try to help release this emotional tension; instead, it promotes it by using suppression measures. And then they're surprised when schizophrenics don't speak about their feelings enough — well, they're forced to lock them up inside themselves.

The test period of a month was coming to a close. The sculptors certified I had "great talent and was exceptionally hard-working." On one of the last days, I was suddenly overcome with an inexplicable fear for Molt while I was at work. Something elusive seemed to be threatening him. Was it the approaching war? Molt wound up in a Russian prison and wasn't released for a long time, as I found out many years later from a mutual friend. But the war hadn't even begun yet. "Save him! Help him!" I prayed in my fear. At this moment the basement doorbell rang. It had never rung down here before. Relieved, I stood up. A sign of being heard? A Roma[1] stood at the door. She took my hand and looked at the lines. "You will succeed at everything." She offered me shampoo powder. I accepted it gratefully.

A sunny morning in the first week of July. In the afternoon, the singer wanted to visit me to choose a sculpture. But I had the urge to leave the studio. I bicycled out of town. For four weeks I'd worked in the basement from morning till the late afternoon. Now I had to get out. I lay down in a field of grain. Above me was the blue sky with clouds rolling by. I fell asleep. A rainstorm woke me up. I got up. I left my bicycle lying there. I don't know any more whether it seemed too risky to ride my bike during a storm, whether I feared the metal tubing could attract lightning, or whether I planned to get the bike later. I think it had more to do with the feeling of liberation

1 Here Buck uses the German *Zigeunerin,* the term then used for a member of the Roma or Sinti communities and now understood to be a slur.

the psychotic break was setting off: to let go of things, to need nothing more, not to plan or want anything, to simply submit to the inner impulses.

And so I'd overslept the singer's visit in the studio. I walked through the pouring rain. When I saw a telephone booth on the way, I called him. "I bicycled out this morning and fell asleep in a field of grain. Now the storm has taken me by surprise and I got very wet." He laughed: "And I was in the studio." — "Can't you come get me with your car here?" I asked. I never would have thought to ask him something like that under normal circumstances. And on top of that I didn't even know exactly where I was. "Did you choose a sculpture?" I asked him — "Yes." — "But it still needs to be fired." — "Where can you have it fired? At home in the oven?" — "No, that won't work." — "And when are you coming for your singing lesson?" — "When I think of it, I'll come." I wanted to appear to him just through my thoughts — just as he and Molt had appeared to me at the crossing in Halle. Because I still believed that this hallucination had been a result of Molt's thinking of me.

I returned to the town in the pouring rain. A bicyclist got off his bike and walked by my side. "What do you know?" — "A lot," I said and made a knowing face, although I still didn't know more about what he meant than I'd read in the home economics encyclopedia.

That night, the stairs creaked. My friend and her fellow students had already left for the break or an internship. I heard people speaking quietly above my room. The old gentleman in the room of his housekeeper! He seemed to me to be very old at the age of seventy. At this age, I had thought one would only engage in platonic relationships. When my friend was here, I had never heard him.

The next morning, I didn't go into the studio but far away toward town. By the bank of a little lake or expanded river I sat down and sang my Rilke songs and whatever melodies I thought of to go with poems. Here, where I thought myself alone, I sang as loudly as I could. An old bent man appeared from over the embankment. "What on earth are you doing there?" he called to me. "I am singing," I yelled back and walked toward him. Behind the embankment there was a little power station which he apparently operated by himself. "May I make a telephone call here?" I asked. —"Who do you want to call?"—"I want to ask a friend to pick me up."

We walked over to the station. The man opened the door of the telephone booth and banged it shut behind me. It seemed a little strange to me and somewhat creepy. In the telephone book I looked for Molt's name. Nobody answered. "Is your friend going to pick you up?" the man asked when I came out of the booth. "Yes, he's coming." We walked outside. "See, there he is already." A VW was turning into the street in front of us and stopped at some distance. I walked over to it. A painter, who had just unpacked his watercolor pad, sat inside. He actually resembled Molt a little, it seemed to me. "When are you leaving?" I asked. He had actually intended to paint, he said. But he opened the car door and offered me a cigarette, which I hardly knew how to smoke properly. We talked about Worpswede, which I had experienced that previous fall with my friend.—"Where do you want to drive?" I gave him Molt's address and he drove me back to town. He stopped in front of a hair salon by a plaza close to a church, got out and opened the car door. I thanked him and walked into the store without looking at the house number. "Do the Molts live here?" "They don't live here anymore," the barber said, "they moved." I stared at the back of the man's head whose hair he was cutting. Didn't it look just like the back of Molt's head? Was Molt sitting right there in front of me staying silent, letting the barber talk in his stead? "They don't live here anymore!" the barber repeated.

I left the store and wandered through the shopping streets. In a bookstore I asked for a cookbook and a book about gymnastics. During the first singing weekend, Mrs. Molt did morning gymnastics with us. I took the thickest of the cookbooks. I didn't have any money on me. Nonetheless, the bookseller packed both the books and gave them to me. Whomever do you want to cook for without a husband and children? I asked myself as I walked through the street and threw the package into an open basement window. Later I received a receipt that was marked as paid.

In one store I looked at typewriters although I didn't know how to type. In another store punchbowls — the vessels for parties. Finally, I asked to see wedding rings at a jeweler's. "These please!" I didn't even try them on. The messenger would deliver the rings.

In front of the old gentleman's house, I ran into the messenger. I pulled the smaller ring over my finger and then gave it back to the messenger. The name still had to be engraved, I said, and told him Molt's first name. But that would have to happen today. "Because this evening I'm going to Heligoland." The messenger looked at me in a panic. It was the same opaque look I'd seen two years ago from the employee in the hospital in A. when I called Molt.

Why had I said that? I had no intention of going to Heligoland. How would I even have gotten there? My mouth said the words, although I hadn't thought of Heligoland even for a second. But I also had no intention of buying the ring. It was enough to have had it on my finger briefly and given the instructions to have Molt's name engraved on it. It was a symbolic act to calm me down. Because the certainty I'd derived from the gypsy's words had left quickly. The cookbook and the gymnastics book, the punch bowl and the typewriter, had also been symbols. A dark feeling told me that I would someday need the typewriter. Because what erupted forcefully in the laundry room that morning of the first break now filled me again with a quiet certainty: one day I would have something to say. And the approaching war was now a certainty again, even if I did not have the thought that I could stop it.

The messenger got on his bicycle. She's crazy!, his scared expression told me. I went inside the house.

I ate something and left, walking toward the zoo. In the weeks of my workaholic phase I had never gone to see it. I didn't want to stay inside the house. In particular, I did not want to stay the night here. I put on my jacket, the night was going to be chilly. I wandered about aimlessly through the dusky streets with their gardens out front. It grew dark. How about if I went to see the singer? Since I had been sterilized, I had suppressed any thought of loving a man. Love wouldn't be possible for me. All the men I knew wanted to get married and have children. Aside from which, it was illegal to marry someone who was sterilized. To live with a man out of wedlock back then would have been impossible. Later I heard from a forcibly sterilized woman who'd married after 1945 that she had to listen to accusations about her sterilization during a marital argument. The exclusively negative evaluation of psychosis by psychiatry makes us the victims of the superior thinking of "normal people."

I felt unmistakably drawn to the singer who was twenty years older than me. He expressed feelings in his singing which were otherwise not uttered. The sound of his voice and his vital, feeling rendition let one feel human warmth and space; that this was quietly accompanied by something unleashed seemed soothing to me.

I needed this natural, unpretentious human being. And now I would go to him, I suddenly decided resolutely. I was filled with a joyous tension. I took off the silver wristwatch I'd gotten for my confirmation and threw it over the fence of a front garden. What did I still need a watch for? The inner impulses had broken out again, I could simply follow them. Then I took off my blue velvet jacket and threw it over another front yard fence. I felt as if I was on my way to him, with flowing hair. Would I also have dared ringing his doorbell? Probably not. "But my dear child, so late at night you are coming to visit me?" He would have probably been embarrassed. But my steps didn't even lead me to his street. He would hardly have been in his town apartment anyway; he was probably in his house far away from the town, in which his family lived in summer.

A man was walking next to me. He took my hand. "But it's very cold!" He put it in his jacket pocket and warmed it up. I let it happen wordlessly. "I'll make you some hot coffee upstairs in my room," he said. Silently I went upstairs with him. He unlocked his door: a spacious, but, in its lack of personality, depressing rented room. Above the rectangular table a lamp with a green glass shade was on, behind it a plush sofa. On the wall opposite me a large colorful picture hung over the bed: a red rock island in the ocean — Heligoland! That is why my mouth had told the messenger: "This evening I'm going to Heligoland."

I remained standing close to the door but was not afraid. The man brewed the coffee and poured it from the thermos into the cup. His movements and his words seemed self-conscious. A person who lived under the pressure of his superiors, it seemed to me. I didn't even put the cup into my hand by myself; he had to bring it to my mouth. I didn't move and didn't speak but the joy still filled me. "I will warm you up," the man said and hugged me. But I could see that he felt uncomfortable seeing me standing there silently, motionless and filled with joy.

He took me downstairs in front of the house. I sat down on the stoop of the house door. He went upstairs. After a while he came back. "Please go!" he said. I remained seated. He went upstairs but came back down soon thereafter. "Please just go!" I remained seated silently. Where was I supposed to go? I didn't know. I didn't want to go back to the house of the old gentleman, and I didn't even have the house keys. The man came downstairs again and asked me to leave. Finally, a police car arrived and took me to the station. The next morning, I was taken to the institution that was just outside of the town. My second institution.

This time I was relieved: in the institution there was absolutely nothing I could do to stop the war that was coming. Ilten was a private second-class institution and was more like a sanatarium.[2] Everything that had frightened and confused me ever more deeply in the "restless ward" in Bethel didn't exist here: no duration baths, no wet applications, no cold showers on the head, no stinking paraldehyde, no narcotic injections, no belts on the bed. And no Bible quotes, which had just intensified my confusion because inhumane things were happening underneath them. Additionally, the patients weren't constantly lying in their beds. There was no restless ward one could be transferred to as punishment. When I threw my washbasin to the floor in a rage one morning so that it broke, I heard no words of reproach.

Now my rage was directed toward England. That had to do with the approaching war I again believed was about to begin. That it should have been England in particular that perturbed me probably came from a lighter patch of skin on my right hip, whose form had reminded me of the British Isle; because of that I felt a closer attachment than to other countries. I literally carried it on my skin.

My memories of the three months in Ilten are weaker than those during my time in Bethel; everything was too normal here for it to leave a deeper impression. There were no large halls but instead four beds to a room; later I was moved to a two-bedroom in an open ward. I lived alone there; the windows could be opened all the way. There also were no locked faucets; every patient had her own washing station with a porcelain washbasin. Everything was so normal here that I initially had difficulties

2 Such an institution would be more focused on convalescence.

believing it. When an older nurse accompanied me into the large park, a long one-story building with many doors made me suspicious. What could be behind those doors? After the experiences in Bethel, I simply couldn't imagine that there wasn't something else hidden behind the friendly surface.

I wrote the singer a letter; I warned him of the approaching war and added that he might think of something to hinder the war. Because I could think of nothing and anyway, I was stuck here.

I took the letter to the mailbox in front of the gate of the institution park. That the gate wasn't locked was as surprising to me as everything else here. So that's how richer patients experienced an institution. My aunt who was paying for my stay wrote to me shortly before I was discharged: "That you preferred being in Ilten so much more than Bethel must have also contributed to your faster recovery."

The only thing I was very frightened of here were the cardiazol[3] injections. In the morning before breakfast, the old professor who directed the institution would inject me in the arm. I felt the spasming liquid flow through my veins because during the entire procedure I did not become unconscious. It was very torturous. The injections were actually supposed to make one unconscious, because the intention was to artificially induce spasming and unconsciousness through cardiazol, insulin, or electroshocks; this questionable method had been developed after doctors observed that epilepsy and schizophrenia didn't occur in the same individual.[4]

Aside from these injections, however, I don't remember anything unpleasant. I made friends with a thirteenth-grader and ran about the large, unlocked institution park

3 These injections were an older form of current Electro-Convulsive Therapy, or ECT. Both are intended to induce grand mal seizures.

4 Not true, of course.

with her. We sat with the aristocratic female gardener, a former patient, in front of the greenhouse. So that's how one transplants plants. She showed us. We talked about music. For the first time since my sterilization, I could feel like a totally normal being again. I was even able to engage in being silly. We stepped over the low fence of the pony pasture and braided the ponies' tails together as they grazed next to one another.

When second class became too expensive, I lived in a simple two-bedroom on the first floor of an also open house of the third class[5] for the rest of my time. Here too, we were able to open the windows completely. I was also allowed to move about freely, still remember the fields of grain and the pastures surrounded by hedges. There were no locked-up maintenance patients as in Bethel. The long-term patients worked during the day with the farmers in the village and didn't return until the afternoon. My roommate was a woman about forty years old who was unable to walk. She sat in front of a pillow and made lace. Her face glowed from within. This sweet face of a person who had turned inward completely because of their walking disability still stands out for me very clearly.

The warmhearted female doctor had told me about this woman and said I was sure to feel comfortable with her. That too was different here: the doctors spoke with us. But even here, I was not asked about my psychosis experience and its history.

It was said that the directing professor had many years prior married a patient. Clearly, he did not consider us inferior human beings. Ilten for the most part assimilated one to normal life and so let us experience how helpful it was for patients not to be locked up and not to be devalued. The trust as well that was demonstrated to us in the form of unlocked doors and windows that could be

5 Tiers of care based on pay was not unusual in Germany at this time.

opened gave us a sense of well-being; we couldn't disappoint this trust. We were peaceful even without psychotropic drugs,[6] which didn't enter the market for fifteen more years. Nowadays, psychiatrists like to praise wards that have become quiet due to psychotropic drugs. But that is anything but a recommendation for them. Well-directed institutions and wards that don't hold patients without giving them something to do were quiet as well, before the advent of psychotropic drugs. There were no "raging" patients in Ilten who grew more aggressive and in whatever way more confused.

Nobody bashed their heads against the walls out of bitterness the way Mrs. Pastor did in Bethel. I did not see such serious symptoms in any of my later institutions than I experienced there—neither my own nor in patients around me. The normal environment and the friendly treatment in Ilten couldn't promote or strengthen psychotic ideas as did the "restless ward" in Bethel, which was hermetically sealed and locked away from the outer world. That ward had provoked them in such a terrifying way. That is probably also why there were fewer sterilization applications than in Bethel.

And this patient-friendly institution in the year 1938—one year before the start of the euthanasia murders! Was it because Ilten was a private institution that was supported by stockholders? Presumably we, like our relatives, were considered clients whose needs had to be taken into account. Keeping long-term patients without giving them work to do would have been unprofitable for a stockholding company. The long-term patients of the third class in Ilten were still in a much better situation, because they worked on farms while the patients in the locked wards of the communal and church institutions were generally kept unoccupied and dwindled away. How

6 Chlorpromazine, or Thorazine, was the first widely used antipsychotic and synthesized in 1951.

many of them paid with their lives a year later[7] when they were unable to prove they were capable of working? And how many held patients still are dwindling due to their medications?

Ilten was encouraging for me. How much more moved was I when I recently found in the documentary *Healing and Destroying in the Model Region Hamburg* by Angelika Ebbinghaus, Heidrun Kaupen-Haas, and Karl Heinz Roth[8] a letter from the murder organization Gekrat[9] from November 1941 to the Hamburg health administration: "Based on the agreement you made with our Mr. Siebert we moved 150 ill patients from Hamburg-Langenhorn to the institution Ilten. We kindly ask you to transfer the sum of 2727.80 RM for ensuing expenses and which are listed in the attached invoice to our postal check account in Berlin 29 924."

It says in the paragraph "Moved to [...] and killed." Did Ilten fulfill the function of acting as an intermediary station prior to the final move to an institution, which after gassing ended in 1941, poisoned and let the patients starve?[10]

My second break had subsided, my mother picked me up. In my two breaks the inner impulses had broken out following a spiritual burden; both times I experienced this breaking open as a liberation from the previous burden. In both breaks symbols took on a dominating meaning. The burden was, however, not comparable. In 1936 it

7 Inability to work was one of the main criteria for death in T4. Additionally, Hitler had vowed to rid Germany of schizophrenia.

8 A book with the same title was published in 1991: Angelika Ebbinghaus, Heidrun Kaupen-Haas, and Karl Heinz Roth, *Heilen und Vernichten im Mustergau Hamburg: Bevölkerungs- und Gesundheitspolitik im Dritten Reich* (Hamburg: Konkret-Literatur-Verlag, 1991).

9 Gekrat was part of T4 and operated transportation of victims to killing centers.

10 It was indeed the case that Ilten had served as a holding center, a facility used to house victims temporarily before transport to the killing centers.

was a deep developmental crisis, an inner breakdown and then a desperate attempt over weeks to find a relationship to Jesus. And in spite of the strong connection to Molt, to be able to stand on my own two feet again, independently. The idea of being "the bride of Christ" had overwhelmed me at the time, but I had also been shown a path to develop my own nature. In 1938, a minor impetus, the singer's question, had been enough to trigger the second break.

The singer's question was basically harmless, but it addressed my deep insecurity: I was forcibly sterilized, felt as a "mentally ill woman" that I had a stain and knew from reference books the damning prognoses for schizophrenics. That is why after about three weeks the inner impulses must have had to break out again: with the feeling of being led from within, being accepted by God, they liberated me from this constant spiritual burden. Because of my devaluation as an "unempathetic schizophrenic woman," and the inner isolation, my readiness for psychosis had grown. A small impulse was enough for it to break open again.

6

The Shock

Now followed a good time with my parents in their new home. Nobody here knew that I had come from an institution. When our organ player died in the spring of 1939, Father suggested I learn to play the organ and take over his position. As a part-time organ player with the C-Exam, I would perhaps not be entirely dependent on the perhaps breadless art. I had reservations; I couldn't play piano and so I was missing the foundation. But since I could practice as much as I wanted to, I did learn after all — thanks also to my good (female) organ teacher — and later took over the position.

I met my first boyfriend at the organ. He lived entirely in the music and could express himself directly through improvisation. We were very close and experienced it as painful that we weren't allowed to have more than friendship.

And then the outbreak of the war arrived on September 1, 1939. The young women in our town, myself included, were drafted as munitions workers outside. So, the war had indeed started, even if it came three and a half years after the morning in the laundry room, when I was overcome with the certainty that it was on its way. The question about the nature of schizophrenia thus occupied me anew. Someone who is diagnosed with "schizophrenia" must understand what they experience.

The certainty of the approaching war had overpowered me and found me completely unprepared back then; never before had I thought of the possibility of war. It was similar to the answer to the jeweler's messenger, where I had without a thought claimed I was traveling to Heligoland that evening, although up to that second, I'd never thought of Heligoland; then in the evening I stood in front of the big picture with the red rock island Heligoland—but that too, I could of course not have known beforehand. I thought of both as "epiphanies," which had seemingly broken in from the outside. Were there, maybe, hidden connections that were closed off to the normal consciousness?

Even the simultaneity of events that normal consciousness calls a "coincidence," I experienced as meaningful in a psychotic state: the appearance of the painter in the moment when I tried calling Molt in vain; the gypsy ringing at the basement door the moment I was filled with fear for Molt. The idea that this convergence of events couldn't be a coincidence but meant something made perfect sense. During my last break in 1959, these experiences of a secret connection of meaning were magnified, and I finally recognized in them the decisive characteristic through which the psychotic experience of the world differed from the normal one. The awakening of my instinct that I experienced as a guide from within and which gave me assuredness in my actions that I hadn't had in a normal state, also points to the context beyond conscious thought and volition. As ridiculous as many things may appear that my awakened instinct led me to do—in so doing I felt guided and protected and in this state nothing bad happened to me even in precarious and dangerous situations.

Psychiatry, which calls the psychotic sense-experiencing "delusion" and declares it pathological, doesn't recognize something very essential. It seems to be of immense importance whether the psychotic individual trustingly hands themselves over to the experience of a meaning context closed off to the normal experience of the world; this experience probably only seems destructive to someone who is overcome by fear and panic. That is why it is so fatal for the patient when their experiences are declared pathological and meaningless, so that their value as a human being is questioned. But all of that was in no way clear to me toward the end of 1939.

The very end of 1939, I was released from my work in the munitions factory and could continue my vocational training. In May of 1941, I passed the minor organ exam and subsequently started my training as a sculptor. Since we weren't sure whether I would be accepted into an arts academy as a sterilized woman, I attended a private art school for a year. I lived with my aunt. My uncle had been thrown into jail by the Nazis for "subversive actions against the state." We were waiting for his letters, waiting for my aunt to be allowed to speak to him. Waiting for army mail from my cousins, my brother, my friend. In February of 1942, my brother died from the effects of an injury. My parents had been able to see him in the military hospital a week earlier and had been full of hope, because for a time he couldn't return to the Russian front.

In our quarter there was a relatively large number of Jewish families, a few lived in our apartment building. But what does one know about one another in a big city? On both the Christian and the Jewish side, relatively little had been done to encourage neighborly contact; here they were limited to saying hello. Very early one morning at the end of the summer of 1942, I saw four or five Jews standing on a square close by with suitcases and next to them two civilians without suitcases and without a yellow star. It was obvious that they had been ordered here to be picked up in a discrete way. Where to, nobody knew.

The inhumane happened silently beside the commonplace. My friend's parents—he a renowned painter, she a former student of his—mentioned the sermon the bishop of Galen[1] had given in the cathedral on August 3, 1941; printed copies were distributed. Why I didn't read this call to conscience back then, and only twenty years later found out about the transport of eight hundred patients from the Institution Warstein to their death, I don't know anymore.

In the mornings, we sculpted nudes using models; in the afternoon my two friends and I sculpted the portrait of a twelve-year-old girl. The critique twice a week didn't satisfy us. But the artistic suggestions by friends gave me a lot. Through them I also learned about the works of the artists being defamed as "degenerate." My friend's father had painted portraits of many of them: Käthe Kollwitz, Emil Nolde, Ernst Barlach, and others. Even in the loo, the most beautiful pictures hung above one another; here one could take one's time looking at them. My untiring parents sent potatoes and other food that was in especially short supply in the major cities.

I registered with the Frankfurt Academy of Art in the winter semester of 1942. The entry exam took fourteen days: nature drawing, sculpting a portrait, and a composition of choice on the topic "Sculpture and Architecture." After passing the exam, one had to take a medical exam. Mother wrote: "Now you will hopefully be successful in answering all questions truthfully without feeling constrained. Of course that's not that easy since you always are worried that your illness could upset your plans. That is why we are especially happy and grateful that you are taking it easy... 'To persist against all odds,' I must think of this Goethe quote constantly today."

I took it "calmly" because my professor overseeing the exam appreciated my design for the exam task "Sculpture and Architecture." I designed a round concert hall. The

1 Sermons by the Catholic bishop Clemens August Graf Von Galen against Aktion T4 were instrumental in its official end, which also resulted in the move to wild euthanasia.

podium for the musicians was pushed into the audience space, and in the outer walkabout I sketched six listening figures in the recesses in the wall. The figures were seated, but the closer they got to the concert podium, the more they stretched to hear with an upward momentum. I was sure that at the art academy there were other measures than those used by doctors. But which ones decided one's acceptance? There I was not so sure.

I was lucky. The physical exam only went as far as the belt. I only remember my fear that my sterilization scar would be discovered, and I would lose my acceptance. I definitely would have answered the question about earlier operations in the negative. But I don't think I was asked about that. A fellow applicant who came from the Munich Academy was rejected because she wasn't Aryan. The professor because of whom, like me, she had come to Frankfurt, wanted to accept her but he had no choice. He had nothing to do with Nazi ideology. She returned to Munich. I felt she drew the best horse head and sculpted the best portrait.

I went to the class for live model drawing; I really missed it. We drew with charcoal and in a large format, using live models. I wanted to be able to sculpt my model drawings and so I covered them in a whole net of lines that followed the forms; this kind of drawing had impressed me with the animal sculptor Philipp Harth. The professor at first stood in front of the pages that were covered in hatching somewhat baffled; as a painter, light and shadow sufficed for him. But for me precisely understanding form was important. During general evening figure drawing, with frequent position changes, I recovered from the project drawing of the day and only pursued sketching. "The appeal of your drawings lies in how you keep breaking the forms," one of my painting class colleagues said. He belonged to the group of soldiers who were given time off to study one or two semesters. We female students sometimes spent days at a time helping families with children.

The colleague showed me his pictures and gave me his fairytales to read. Now we spoke more frequently about what occupied and moved us. We couldn't accept that the hell of the here and now should continue in the afterlife, with a renewed split of humanity into heaven and hell, but exactly the other way around: "eternal life" for the "righteous" and for the others "eternal torment." That didn't seem to be compatible with love.

That was the winter of 1942–43 when the hell of Stalingrad happened. We learned little about the hell in our own country, about the bomb raids on almost all the major cities. Jochen Klepper had committed suicide with his Jewish wife in 1942, as did the thirty-four-year-old Hugo Distler.[2] His polyphonic choral movements had left a deep impression on me.

A colleague thought Jesus should not have allowed a premature end to his own life. He should have shown us by example what it was to live life with all our human problems, he felt. Being married. Getting old. As a soldier he had experienced a lot of shocks that triggered many questions. My main problem remained the sterilization. Bethel had taken me by surprise, it had turned itself into our judge. This judgment so little convinced me that Jesus's role as judge of the world in the Last Judgment had become questionable to me. A loving father would hardly let his son, even if he was his favorite, judge his children. He would let everyone recognize by themselves whom they hadn't helped but had instead harmed.

A month earlier, my good friend wrote me happily that he had found the girl who was going to become his

2 Jochen Klepper was a German writer and journalist. Denied visas to leave the country, he, his wife, and his daughter committed suicide together. Hugo Distler was a German organist and composer who committed suicide at thirty-four, partly due to fear of conscription into the German army.

wife. He asked me to remain his best female friend. That appeared more difficult to me than the temporary ending of our friendship. But the separation was difficult and stirred up a lot in me. At the time I wrote a number of poems. One of them went like this:

Dandelion

As the sun's embers stopped glowing
and the moon blossomed, too round and soft
a spray of seeds fell on the earth
and from it grew dandelion.
Dandelion, touch me,
that from your seedball
just one ray
fall in my soul as well.
That I glow like the sun
that I blossom, blossom, blossom
little dandelion.

That when sorrow closes my blossom
in the night
dark, gently,
I guard the blossom.

Dandelion, touch me,
that from blossom comes seed,
round and soft,
like the moon,
and I once as the most wonderful reward
drift in front of God's throne.
Help me do that, amen.

As the sun's embers stopped glowing
and the moon blossomed, too round and soft
a spray of seeds fell on the earth
and from it grew dandelion.

The winter semester came to a close. In our conversations, I felt directly connected to my colleague. So much more heavily was my soul weighed down by being shut out from love and feeling the inner isolation of a mentally ill woman. I could speak with no one about my psychotic experiences that I felt as so much a part of me, even if I could not explain where they came from. And once again the psychosis liberated me from the isolation. Again, the feeling of secret, incomprehensible contexts broke out that I didn't experience in a normal state.

One day and one night I strayed about aimlessly. The thought of suicide had helped me continue to live after the sterilization; the morning after this straying March night I actually attempted suicide for the first time. Making a spontaneous decision I jumped from the middle of a bridge over the Main in my heavy winter coat. I sank to the ground, resurfaced, and now decided death by drowning was actually quite unbearable. I couldn't swim well but I gathered all my strength and reached the bank. An ambulance took me to the university psych ward.

From the end of March until the beginning of June 1943 I experienced this clinic with its friendly nurses. The director at the time was Professor Karl Kleist. According to Alice von Platen-Hallermund's report about Hessian euthanasia institutions (*The Killing of the Mentally Ill in Germany*, 1948[3]), Kleist was the only psychiatric professor besides Professor Ewald in Göttingen who opposed killing patients. Silently Kleist went through the main ward and a few smaller rooms. But the attitude of the nurses implied their instruction was friendly toward patients.

In the mornings we pulled horsehair, which was used to fill mattresses back then — monotonous work but better than none. And unlike in Bethel, visitors were allowed

3 Alice Platen-Hallermund, *Die Tötung Geisteskranker in Deutschland* (Frankfurt am Main: Verlag der Frankfurter Hefte, 1948). This publication was reprinted in 1993 by Psychiatrie-Verlag in Bonn.

in the day room of our ward. My mother came right away; later my classmates and our model did as well. This ward with newly admitted and dischargeable patients made a quiet impression — even without medication-induced suppression.

During a consultation in the doctor's room, the first thing I did was grab a syringe lying on the desk and throw it against the wall where it shattered. "Why did you do that?" the ward doctor asked. He said it in an interested manner and without any kind of reproach. "It was a symbolic act," I explained to him. That a psychiatrist should ask about the motivation for an action was quite new to me. Yet he did not ask about the meaning of the action. Perhaps he guessed it.

After just about four weeks I was subjected to a four-week insulin cure. One would think that a "cure," as it was officially called, would be something healing. But it was a torturous procedure that only suppressed via medication, instead of healing. Before breakfast insulin was injected, every morning a little more. Not quickly as with the sedative injection, but bit by bit for hours we grew weaker; we broke out in sweat and became restless. I was so weak that I kept letting my head fall from one side of the pillow to the other until I finally fell into a coma. Every time it was like a slow death, day in, day out, for four weeks. We were brought back to consciousness with very sweet peppermint tea that was infused into us through a nasal probe. Then there was lots of buttered bread for a late breakfast.

It was more difficult every day to remember anything, after waking up from the coma. Normal things slipped my mind as much as psychotic ones. But I didn't want to forget my experiences under any circumstances. The daily unconsciousness made it ever more difficult. The instinct that had broken out became ever weaker. That was what the procedure was meant to do. But this has nothing to do with healing. To be healed one must understand and process what one has experienced. Here it was just massively repressed and the suppressed then had to surface during the next break.

I wrote my mother that this suppression cure couldn't heal me. She answered: "Beloved child, of course we know that it will be hard for you but you simply must trust the doctor... Just surrender completely to the hands of the experienced doctors and the sooner you will get well again. Even ten years ago this didn't exist yet." Two weeks later she wrote: "We believe that you need to have the attitude that as a layperson you cannot judge it and that the best and smartest thing to do is to trust the doctor who you know is capable."

I could hardly consider myself a layperson anymore. I had experienced my psychoses much too consciously for that. I knew their spiritual backstories; the opinion of Professor Kleist and his doctors that it was an "endogenous" psychosis, in other words, a physically induced event whose spiritual side effects were meaningless, couldn't convince me. That five years after the suppression with Cardiazol shocks in Ilten this new break had surfaced proved that suppression didn't really help. And how could it have helped? I considered the psychosis a meaningful, if also difficult to understand, experience, and only understanding could have helped in that situation. Over the next sixteen years I experienced two more breaks, the next one just three years after the suppression through insulin in Frankfurt. During the last breaks I was able to make observations in myself and a fellow female patient that became significant in understanding my psychosis and finding healing.

Following the insulin cure, we helped the female doctor infuse the sweetened tea via a nasal probe into our fellow female patients. One of these patients, who was around my age, did not respond to the cure as well as expected. It was very difficult for her to orient herself upon waking up from the coma. The doctor made a regretful comment that "it was too bad about her." Why too bad about her, we wondered. What could this mean? Apparently, none of us ever thought our psychotic experiences could make someone feel sorry for us; it was much too fundamental an experience for us to even consider this. An old, local female patient later took me aside and quietly said: "She will be transferred to 'Eichberg.'" And she alluded to the fact that "Eichberg" let its patients go hungry, perhaps even let them starve to death. I couldn't believe that. Only twenty years later did I find out through the sparse euthanasia literature and the editorial of a former Eichberg patient that she'd been right about what she whispered.

The Frankfurt university hospital was renowned at the time, but it was impossible to think their understanding of psychosis was based on actual research. One reduced oneself to the observation of symptoms; no one asked about our psychosis experience and patient history. Psychoses were considered "endogenous" somatic episodes; conversations about their content and their genesis seemed superfluous. Even when patients were presented to students during seminars, it happened without first talking to us.

I was facing such an involuntary presentation. What the professor or the chief physician was trying to make the students understand was a mystery, because he neither knew my history nor the motives for my suicide attempt. I wrote to my father beseechingly, but he only received my second letter; the first one was held back by hospital censor — a practice which to the present day goes against the constitution, as I have read in Frank Fischer's book *Insane Asylums: Patients Accuse.*[4] My father really tried his best on my behalf back then. He wrote to the professor and urgently asked him to desist from presenting me because

4 Frank Fischer, *Irrenhäuser: Kranke klagen an* (Munich: Kurt Desch, 1969).

it could impact my further studies; he also offered to pay the higher cost of second class if that made stopping the presentation easier. The chief physician phoned from the lecture hall to the ward that I was to be tied to the gurney in the event I resisted. But the ward doctor hid me in a broom closet. I really appreciated him for that. Maybe he also had a guilty conscience because of the letter he'd held back. The presentation would have been especially bad for me because the lectures were visited by students from the art academy, including ones from my class.

It felt good that my parents really stood by me in this situation. In Bethel I'd felt left alone and abandoned by my parents during the first eleven weeks until my mother visited the first time. But why had they internalized the medical opinion that my psychosis had a physical cause? This I couldn't understand. They knew about my conversations with Molt and my long letter to him and experienced my reaction to his response. During her first visit to Bethel, Mother even told the chief physician that my psychosis had probably been triggered by a spiritual shock, which the latter, however, didn't accept. I've often asked myself whether they wouldn't have been able to understand my psychosis experiences if we'd had a conversation about them. Since the Bible is full of symbols and symbolic acts, and even baptism and holy communion are symbolic acts, shouldn't my father have understood me as a theologian? But attempts at conversation failed because my parents trusted the opinions of doctors. They would have gone along with the opinions of a psychotherapist who understood my psychosis just as matter-of-factly. But these psychotherapists didn't exist.

Psychiatrists have no idea how much alienation they bring to families with their dogma of somatic episodes. If the patient's experience is reduced to being "meaningless"—how should that keep from damaging contact with their next of kin? Among the files that my father saved, I found a 1936 evaluation from Bethel that certified my "permanent inability to work due to a mental defect." Apparently, the chief physician had been asked to certify this and couldn't subsequently say anything else when asked by the genetic health court—this is how I read the document. It really hurt me that my parents had so little trust in me. I asked them in a letter whether they still considered me "fit for life" since I interpreted "permanent" to mean "for life." Had they needed the evaluation to continue receiving the childcare cost in spite of my interrupted vocational training? I felt quite a bit of bad feeling and resentment around this issue. It wouldn't have been necessary if the psychotic wasn't written off as a person whose experiences and reactions were determined by a physical defect, and so were meaningless and unworthy of empathy.

But more significant was the fact that I couldn't engage in a conversation about my psychosis with my parents. I'd tried from Frankfurt. Mother initially answered: "Unfortunately I have no time these days and the long letter should be answered in a quiet moment. But you should know how happy we are that you gave us your insights into what moved you." At least she reassured my worry that my parents might not consider me "fit for life": "After all, you have achieved something and we are absolutely convinced that you will be able to earn your keep." It took three weeks for a more comprehensive response, but it also proved how strongly the psychiatric dogma influences the family. I will quote longer passages to illustrate this. Mother wrote:

> We are still processing your letter and I wish I were with you so we could talk about all of this in person. We really want to visit but preferably not till next week....
>
> Now I want to try to write in a way that will really make us understand one another. I am so sorry that we did you wrong with our worry that you might have made critical remarks regarding other patients.... Isn't

that right, that you shouldn't be angry, if parents worry their child might have done something wrong, to warn them.

We must have not received one of your letters because we do not have the one in which you complained about Dr. N. That is why we didn't know about your worry that your case would be presented in the lecture hall, otherwise Father would have written right away. He was probably held back by the testing nurse because of this complaint. And one must show understanding for this.... Because when they are sick, patients often wrong their doctors and then take it back when they can see clearly again. Then it is often better that their utterances don't reach their families, who of course get very upset about such things....

My dear child, the sterilization happened entirely without our support. It was so difficult for us, I can't even express it and we were so worried how it would affect you. But we were entirely powerless. I still remember how Dr. St. [the doctor in Mother's native town whom we visited the beginning of April 1936] wrote to us: there is nothing but resignation in this situation. And of course it's not just one doctor who makes this decision but a court. That is why there was such hesitation to put you in an institution because one was afraid that this would happen. I often told myself later: we shouldn't have waited so long until there was the catastrophe in..., but that was the reason. In Bethel they were very careful before calling the illness by its name. This was preceded by examinations that went for weeks. I myself was there when the case was being tried in court. When I asked if there was any way to stop it, one of the gentlemen said: the only one was to have her stay in the institution until she was forty-five. I remember that I said: that's much more terrible. Back then we suffered a lot on your behalf. You didn't notice it perhaps and we avoided letting you see. Perhaps that

> wasn't quite right and you saw it as lacking empathy on our part, and that is why I am actually very happy that this situation is being addressed, because that is how in the end the feeling of alienation arose in you that you wrote about. Perhaps you suffered much more from all of this than we knew. But we really were under the impression that you were taking on this whole weight of life relatively easily and that your life was becoming rich and beautiful through art for which we were time and again grateful from the bottom of our hearts and so we told ourselves: we want to support it as much as we can.

Then there follow passages about the Bethel evaluation: "We don't even remember whether such an evaluation exists.... Because of you, after all, we had to leave... because you were not supposed to return there. That was also only possible because of your illness and the authorities had to do that." The last sentence goes like this: "And isn't it right, my beloved child, now we understand one another better, don't we."

The care in Mother's letter shows that it wasn't a lack of willingness to understand that prevented her, rather, her unwavering trust in the doctors. And that's what caused our alienation and my inner isolation. It wasn't about my wanting more sympathy regarding my sterilization. There was little in my life that was more important to me than my psychosis experience of inner guidance and the closer connection to the whole; in this I found the trust in God that Mother had talked about so frequently. But for my parents, my symbolic rebirth had simply remained a "catastrophe." There were enough other shared experiences between my parents and me—their warm and active participation in my life and their understanding help with my education. But I gave up the attempt to try at an understanding regarding my psychosis following this letter.

What I felt from my parents as a too-fatalistic acceptance of my "mental ailment" and a lack of trust can probably be interpreted as helplessness toward medical authority. Thus the patient who is cheated out of real help from psychiatry is also abandoned by their family.

In her unshakeable trust in the doctors, my unwitting mother also believed that the examinations in Bethel had been comprehensive. The "examinations that went for weeks" could only have been foolish reaction tests; I hadn't noticed any other examinations during the brief daily rounds. I'd felt the chief physician's hug on the mattress as a test of my reaction, and also the strange way he and the female assistant doctor had positioned themselves on either side of my bed like guard soldiers. My resistance to the hug was probably evaluated as "negativistic," my laughter as I shook my head at their strange positions perhaps as "ridiculous," for the assistant doctor said: "It is perhaps much more serious than you think." In this undignified manner diagnoses and sterilization requests had been the result, where instead we needed comprehensive dialogue to reach understanding.

The "fully updated" 7th edition of the *Textbook of Mental and Neurological Illness Care* published in 1975 by Bethel still reads in the section about schizophrenia and its symptoms: "The negativistic sick person doesn't do what one expects of them but rather the exact opposite."[5] But how could we react other than with rejection when being reduced to sheer objects of safekeeping and observation? If the refusal of the patient to fulfill the expectation of doctors during these subjective and completely random "examinations," which are then declared an objective symptom of illness, that must justify a question the other way around: is the psychiatric examination and

5 Karsten Jaspersen, *Lehrbuch der Geistes- und Nervenkrankenpflege*, 7th ed. (Bethel bei Bielefeld: Verlagshandlung der Anstalt Bethel, 1975), 57.

treatment method so inappropriately taken from general medicine a symptom of the negativistic attitude of doctors? Because they refuse to fulfill our justified expectation for understanding and real help, a failure that's in no way random.

The Frankfurt chief physician and later professor Karl Leonhard at least recognized how understandable the patients' negative reactions are. In his *Fundamentals of Psychiatry* from 1948 he wrote: "Indeed, nowadays one has grown accustomed to referring to simple dismissal as negativism. Subsequently one understandably finds the symptom very frequently."[6] But he goes on to say that to keep negativism as a symptom in "its pure form," a doctor would first have to make patients "shift into a friendly mood by talking empathetically with them and in one or the other form winning their trust," and only then perform the reaction test. As if the patients wouldn't detect the manipulation in which their trust was gained by trickery, in order to subject them to a demeaning test of their reactions, one that degrades them to the status of a speechless animal!

Since I seemed unchanged in my parents' eyes between breaks, and my suicide attempt could also count as a manic-depressive symptom, the Bethel diagnosis was changed in Frankfurt into "manic-depressive insanity." I was very relieved about that, because I found in the dictionary that manic-depressive insanity, unlike schizophrenia, didn't lead to "disintegration of the personality" and "impoverishment of emotions." How many suicides might already have been triggered just because of the diagnosis of "schizophrenia" and the prognosis connected to it, which was so damning.

Reading the psychiatric literature after I gained my healing, the diagnosis of "schizophrenia" in fact seemed

6 Karl Leonhard, *Grundlagen der Psychiatrie* (Stuttgart: Ferdinand Enke, 1948), 32.

more accurate. According to Eugen Bleuler, the typical symptoms of schizophrenia are the dissolution of normal trains of thought, bizarre thought patterns, connection and concentrations of unrelated things, use of symbols in place of the original term; he sees the foundational symptom as disruptions of association.[7] Understanding these symptoms as the result of being moved or overwhelmed by the unconscious breaking open is simply neglected. This neglect makes it impossible to understand why the schizophrenic, in their changed experience of the world, feels contexts otherwise unfelt, and almost unavoidably has associations that appear absurd to the normal consciousness. Without these changes in the world context, referred to as "schizophrenic," my close contact with my schizophrenic fellow female patients on a shared symbolic level wouldn't have been possible; the manic-depressive apparently does not experience this connection. That is why the depressive can also accept being called "sick" more easily than the schizophrenic.

Following my cure, I found in the *Fundamentals of Psychiatry* a significant example of how psychiatry tries to prove that "endogenous psychoses" are genetic. Leonhard writes: "Other reasons than the genetic take a step back relative to endogenous psychoses. Following the experiences of war, mental shock does not seem to be a favoring factor for the presentation of schizophrenia."[8] The kind of war experiences we're talking about is described in Hermann Dobbelstein's book *Der normale Mensch im Urteil der Psychiatrie* (*The Normal Person as Seen by Psychiatry*), published in 1955. There it says:

> Nonetheless, it should be mentioned that the psychiatrist must be careful in judging the influence of en-

7 See Eugen Bleuler, *Dementia Praecox oder Gruppe der Schizophrenien* (Leipzig: Deuticke, 1911).

8 Leonhard, *Grundlagen der Psychiatrie*, 87.

> vironmental factors relative to a person. It is a matter of course that they more or less openly contradict psychiatric laypeople who have a different opinion. For example, it may be bitter for the mentally ill person's family to find out that immense mental stress does not cause a real psychosis, but the experiences speak for themselves: in two world wars the number of truly mentally ill people in countries all over the world compared with peacetimes remained about the same.

Even the statistical approach in this line of reasoning is questionable. The patients' own experiences are simply ignored; the content of the psychosis and the connection with their history aren't even taken into consideration. When one has consciously experienced the triggering reason and the development of one's psychosis and can compare these with the reaction to a life-threatening episode in a war, one recognizes the mistake immediately: vital stress is being mistaken for mental stress, in the actual sense of the word.

In 1944, I was squatting under the ruins of a house destroyed by explosive bombs, stuck between the boards of a wardrobe that had buffered the crashing cement ceiling of the bomb shelter. It was totally dark; I couldn't move. My reactions were purely vital, this wasn't about anything but survival and not about inner reorientation in a mental crisis. How long would the boards hold? Did we have a chance of getting rescued? If not, what would our death be like? What had happened to my relatives and our friend, with whom I had only just eaten supper?

The shocks that preceded the breaking out of my schizophrenia were completely different. It was an inner conflict that drew all my energies its way, and through this movement inward the breaking out of the otherwise unconscious was triggered — in other words, what one commonly calls psychosis. But in wartime the energies were directed outward; it was about pure survival, and mental conflicts took a backseat. Everyone was subject to the same fate and so formed a community based on that common fate, a safe community in spite of the dangers; by contrast, an inner conflict that triggers schizophrenia must be mastered in solitude and makes one lonely—just like the devaluation as "mentally ill" which follows. Mental stresses that lead to psychosis are probably situated more in the realm of eros than the threat of death. It follows one would expect a recession of schizophrenic episodes in times of war. The question that must be answered is not why there weren't more schizophrenic episodes in wartime than in peacetime, but rather why there were fewer of them. It is probably due to other kinds of mental conflicts that arise, such as conflicts of conscience or pain over the loss of beloved persons.

I was very bothered by the naive mistaking of vital threat with mental stress in its ordinary sense. As a layperson one cannot even imagine a scientist doing that. So the theory of the purely somatic reasons of psychosis was built on the foundation of such imprecise thinking—a thought error with bad consequences. Many paid for it with their lives, many with lifelong isolation, and myself, like countless others, with forcible sterilization. Which other science is allowed such carelessness? When a bridge collapses, the designing engineer and the contractor are liable. But psychiatry was allowed to hold onto a dogmatic mistake with impunity, one whose practical application destroyed many lives.

At the end of March 1943, I'd been admitted to the university nerve clinic in Frankfurt. In the beginning of June I was discharged as "improved." In 1938 in Ilten, my stay had been barely three months; I'd been in Bethel three quarters of a year. But there too my psychosis had receded on its own after about three months, even without Cardiazol and insulin shocks. That is what I glean from the letters of my parents and siblings that mirror my own letters to them.

7

Death Will Pass

Mother picked me up. I had a vacation job as a mail carrier. Newspapers that I delivered in 1943 reported the heaviest bombings to date of Hamburg. I read about the terrible firestorm in which thousands of Hamburg residents — adults and children — burned alive.

The winter semester began in November of 1943. Already by the end of November, heavy bombing destroyed our academy building. We cleared the rubble and tried to gather up the files that lay strewn about on the street. We took long walks to the rubble rooms because the streetcars couldn't ride anymore.

In the new year of 1944, I drew portraits for some residents in a nursing home because we had to find our own models. My former ward doctor even drew a patient. The next time I came to draw, the psychiatric clinic had also been badly damaged by bombs. At the end of January 1944, another academy building in which we met for critique was destroyed. At the end of March, the Städelschule closed temporarily following more heavy bombings.

I traveled to my grandmother and aunt. There I had the bomb shelter incident I mentioned earlier. The alarm had sounded, we'd sat down at the table in the shelter for dinner. A friend of the family had asked if I could sit at her usual place. That saved my life. After we'd just changed places and started eating, the house collapsed over us and buried us under the rubble. It was pitch-dark. Following the thundering detonation of the explosive bomb and the loud roar of the collapsing building, it became unnervingly quiet. The air pressure had whipped me from my chair. There I squatted, stuck and unable to move either hand or foot. Only my aunt's groans interrupted the noiseless silence. She was unconscious. It was probably only a little more than an hour till one could hear the helpers. Time passed much more slowly for me; we didn't know how many nearby buildings had been destroyed and whether anyone was left to help us get out. Our friend must have been dead immediately. The cement ceiling fell on her. My grandmother and my aunt came away with injuries and broken bones, and both were admitted to the hospital.

The willingness to help on the part of friends was overwhelming. My mother also came. Our friend's death affected me. She had joined our family as a childcare giver and stayed for years when we were little. Now she had been helping my grandmother and my aunt. If we hadn't exchanged places, she would have stayed alive; the ceiling would have fallen on me. Death, which after my sterilization had seemed the only option, would now have occurred almost by itself, without my intervention. I was glad to be alive and hardly injured. But even after months I hadn't gotten over the experience. At the beginning of August, Mother wrote: "When daily life resumes it gets more difficult. Back then I was amazed how well you got over it. I think all that love and care really helped."

Later I entered the already started final semester, before the academy was closed in August of 1944. Our sculpting class had been evacuated to a castle. There were five of us — all girls. Each of us used a different balcony or place in the inside of the castle to build a ceramic female vintner. The most fitting figure was supposed to stand on the fountain of the location. A begun, but unsent, letter to my friend from the private art school gives a report of this unforgettable semester. When I wrote it, we had long been conscripted to work:

> Now I must first tell you about the last and most wonderful semester, the first one with T. I will always be grateful to you that you raved about him and I found him that way. How happy I am to have had these 2½ months.... I was only able to come a month later when everything was already in full swing. Whatever was still useful among the rubble had been brought there. But there was hardly more than modeling stands. They had dug a few of T.'s pieces out of the rubble and with each piece and shard they hugged each other with joy. The castle is located on the Rhine and when we stepped out onto the little balcony it flowed in front of us, wide and peacefully, with many small and large freight ships. Behind it a shining red quarry and on our side an oddly walled-in vineyard.... We had literally been commissioned by the city to restore the beautiful old marketplace fountain's statue of Jacob, and because the saint did not appeal to the student leadership, it was to be replaced by a female vintner.
>
> All of us first worked on sketches and then did one in large format. Each of us created something different and the most suitable figure was actually to go on the fountain. Luckily it didn't get that far. I modeled a kneeling figure, which had to have appropriately larger dimensions. She finally grew to life-size and because until shortly before she was to be cast I hadn't considered that the scaffold hadn't grown as she did, I tugged too hard on her and suddenly had half the figure in my arms.

In the private art school, we had only modeled standing figures using live models, as was the norm. This kneeling one I'd built up from a counterpoint, still present from my organ lessons, following my intuition. Now I wanted to try moving the hand a good centimeter to see whether the composition was still right. It wasn't right anymore. That was surprising for me to see in a life-sized figure. I had to change other things so the relationships of the forms to one another were balanced. That was a very important experience for me. After having been marked as a "mentally ill woman," I was still deeply insecure; but here I experienced that my intuition was right and that I could follow it safely. When you have been devalued to the very center of your being you must have experiences that restore your self-confidence. Perhaps my work in sculpture was especially suitable for that. Even later I often found that work moved along well as long as I trusted the more unconscious, intuitive creative impulses, and that I ruined them when I tried to fix them with too much conscious intention. Or that the backside of a sculpture which I hadn't worked on as consciously was better and more fully expressed than the front.

That proved to me that the center of my being could not be ill. In addition to understanding what has happened in psychosis, healing requires the reestablishment of self-confidence, since it has been damaged by the devaluation of being called "mentally ill." It would be much easier for the affected person if psychiatric treatment didn't devalue them in the first place, and they felt understood.

Two of the five of us were conscripted for anti-aircraft resources. This included the youngest, who had started live model drawing class with me. During the soldier drill, her kidneys were damaged badly and she died aged thirty-two. Prior to that she was strong enough to carve wood sculptures for churches. I was delegated to the post office again. In 1945, I worked as a Red Cross helper for a smaller hospital. First, I worked in the isolation ward for infectious diseases; there were patients with malaria, dysentery, diphtheria, and TB. There were three-legged iron holders in front of the rooms that held enamel bowls for washing hands upon leaving. Two women with TB were the worst off, as they lay in their straw mattress crypts next to the disinfection room. The strong odor from next door wafted through the cracks and wouldn't leave the room. Later on, in the men's ward, we had carried the men on gurneys into the air raid shelter and back up. This took up a lot of time because there were a lot of warnings.

During the last days of the war came a back-and-forth of orders, some to defend the town, others to surrender to the approaching Americans. Following a short fight, in the middle of April 1945 the war in our region was over.

My older and my youngest sister had made their way home before the Russians. Our apartment had remained intact, the family was together, or at least, like my sister, out of danger. Back then that meant a lot. It remained difficult to find food to eat and feel satiated. We looked for nettles for lunch. Whoever had a garden, planted potatoes, sowed vegetables. We didn't have a garden but were able to borrow a piece of lawn and turned the soil. Every turn of the spade brought up half a basket of stones. The potato harvest in the fall was much less productive. My sisters rode to a farmer's one day a week to work and in return received vegetables, potatoes, and sugar beets.

A female friend of my parents who lived in the neighborhood rented out a little room to me to work and sleep in. I had a few commissions: portraits of children, a nativity group for a Catholic chapel, and other things. I also sculpted my friend's young wife's head.

The spring of 1946, Zeller Castle showed the exhibit *Liberated Art,* German Expressionists who had been defamed as "degenerate" during the Third Reich. Many young people with backpacks were there. We sat in front of the paintings for hours on the floor and couldn't get enough of them. I sat longest in front of Emil Nolde's shining watercolor seascapes. I was seeing them for the first time.

It seems strange to me today that only in the 1950s can I remember my shock about the crimes in the concentration camps. Did the thin newspapers cover nothing about them back then? One was relieved to have the horror of the war behind one and concentrated on things that were necessary for life and needed to be taken care of at that moment. Many refugees came to our town with just the bare necessities in their suitcases. "15 million people are straying through Germany or have only found a subpar emergency shelter," *ZEIT* reported in its first issue on February 21, 1946. "Refugees from the cities that have been destroyed by bombs, from other occupation zones, or those who have been deported from neighboring countries."[1] That is almost a quarter of the total German population.

Around this time my fourth break happened. An experience from back then makes the uncertainty of relatives throughout the psychiatric evaluation of psychosis especially clear. I had to have my wisdom teeth removed. The surgeon, who had become a long-time friend with whom my parents shared their common rejection of the Nazis, discussed everything with Mother and me. Then Mother sent me from the room. I knew immediately she was going to tell him about my psychotic breaks and wanted to ask him whether the surgery or the anesthesia could trigger a new one. From her perspective it was an understandable concern because she believed in the psychiatrists' explanations. But for me it was embarrassing to be sent out of the room like a child. I knew the background of my psychosis and knew that being cut out of the conversation was much more of a trigger than surgery or anesthesia. Relatives should always talk *with* the affected and not about them.

Once again, the psychosis started with the breaking out of my instincts. I sat and knitted from morning till night

1 *Die Zeit* 1, February 21, 1946, 1. https://www.zeit.de/1946/01/index.

a dark blue pair of boy's trousers from the unraveled wide sleeves of a sweater. I also knitted a children's coat made of brown woven sheep's wool. I have never knitted a pair of trousers and a coat before, but what would have been arduous was easy and seemed to make itself. In a normal state, I would have had to count stitches and measure whether the yarn was enough for the size. I would have had to steer with my head what I now was able to leave to my hands. I had to knit and was certain that both would fit two refugee children, who needed exactly what I was knitting.

In the dawn of the last night — I thought I was already awake — Molt appeared. He had grown gray and seemed very unhappy. I was very startled. He was a Russian prisoner of war but I didn't know that yet. What did the apparition mean? I was very worried.

The dream vision startled me so much that the next evening I absolutely didn't want to sleep in my studio. I thought about whether I could sleep at home. But on that particular evening, the surgeon was sitting with my parents, and I would have had to go through the room to get to the bedroom. After the embarrassing situation in the hospital prior to my surgery, I had no desire to see him again.

With the breaking out of my instincts my sensation for my surroundings, for our landscape had also changed. This particular evening it was eerie. The old myths with their magic ghosts that are associated with them didn't seem random to me. In a panic I left town after having dropped off at a home for refugee children the pair of trousers and the children's coat. I slept in a hollow in the earth on the outskirts of the next town and got on a train first thing in the morning, although I didn't have any money on me. Nobody asked for a ticket during the ride. In Minden I felt an urge to get off and here too there was no ticket control at the barrier, as was customary.

I didn't think about my family worrying about me. That might have been different if my parents had not trusted the medical opinion of the doctors implicitly, which made a conversation impossible.

All I had taken was a skein of green wool; otherwise, I had nothing with me. I traded the skein for a haircut that made a comb superfluous. Carrying a blooming pussy-willow branch, I ran through the forest singing with the strange feeling that Romans and Teutons had fought right here and there was still something one could sense. With the thick skin of the normal state, I would not have had this sensitivity.

Later I walked all night without getting tired or feeling hungry, although I hadn't eaten since leaving home. Never again did I walk such a long way, so fast on foot. In the morning I reached the city which Molt had called home. Where he lived after his move, I did not know. I arrived at the singer's street and found his house destroyed by bombs. The sculptor in whose studio I'd worked died in the wreckage of her house together with her son.

The misery in the destroyed city and among refugees was horrifying. In a grocery store I asked for ten Reichsmark. The female owner gave them to me immediately. I bought two rolls, an unlined writing pad, a pencil, and later a train ticket back to Minden.

The railway station shelter was full of refugees. I drew them. At night we lay crushed against one another on the floor.

The next morning, I rode back to Minden. At the top of a hill at the edge of the forest I encountered a refugee. He was agitated by the events of those times. We spoke a long time, as if we knew each other well. That evening I went down into the village. He stayed in the little shelter hut.

In the second house a couple took me in. There was a photo in the kitchen; the only son, only just grown up. Yes, he had died, they answered my question. He'd died here in the kitchen, died with struggle. It had happened two years ago, I think, but the grief still lay heavy on them. They let me sleep on the couch in the kitchen.

I experienced something odd that night. Something I cannot capture in words. Perhaps that's why I don't anymore have an exact memory of it. We sat together at breakfast in the morning. I would like to draw the son, I said. They nodded in agreement. And said I should stay for lunch. Then they left. I drew the son from the photo, and I had the urge to write what I'd experienced in the night at the bottom of the drawing: "Death, where is your sting? Hell, where is your victory?"[2] (As far as I know these are Brahms's own writing in his requiem — counter to the Catholic requiem text, he was bitter about death). I put the drawing on the kitchen table and left.

Where was I to stay this night? It was the fifth. Where was I supposed to stay at all? I was overcome by loneliness. I'd never been able to talk to anyone about something that was so essential and meaningful, even if I couldn't understand it. My psychosis was considered mentally ill and was only fought against with shocks; to understand psychosis or to even ask about it didn't seem worth the effort from any psychiatrist's viewpoint. Now, too, I had the institution to look forward to with their measures that were only fighting against the causes. In the evening, once it was dark, death in the Weser[3] seemed to be the best solution.

But one doesn't drown that fast. The water was too shallow. I didn't lose the ground under my feet and so I climbed back up to the riverbank. Perhaps I also realized in the water that this wasn't the right path. In a garden hut, I found dry rags in the moonlight and exchanged them for my wet stuff. Then I stood by the street. A ray of

2 1 Corinthians 15:55, which is usually rendered "Where, O death, is your victory? Where, O death, is your sting?"

3 The Weser is a river in Northwest Germany.

light appeared. A police car. They took me to the station. I stayed in jail a number of days on charges of vagrancy.

I may have had the shock of the cold water to thank for my period, which I hadn't had for two years. So, in fact a physically based psychosis, the somatic would say. I have no doubt, that as in every other mental state, physical processes are also a part of a psychosis. But that is by far no reason to think it is meaningless. For us affected ones it is an essential experience that we cannot separate from ourselves as something worthless, without losing something of value. We must understand and integrate it.[4]

When the jail doctor figured out what my scar was, he gave me a choice: Bethel or Gütersloh. I didn't want to go back to Bethel. Without hesitating I decided to go to Gütersloh.[5]

That is how I learned about the then, and probably still, most renowned communal institution, and since I was still affected by the bleak safekeeping in the "restless ward" of Bethel, Gütersloh made a big impression on me. Here was proof that it wasn't about patients' lacking ability but that it was up to the directors and doctors whether to have the sick decline with inactivity or, as is customary today, stay under the fog and the paralyzing effects of medication.

In the Bethel *Textbook of Mental and Nerve Illness Care* of 1975 it says about Gütersloh:

> In 1923 Hermann Simon introduced a consistent work therapy, the 'more active treatment of the ill in the asylum.' Simon created work opportunities in the institution with a graduated scheme of difficulty. Led in a strict top-down way and with the immense effort of all the institution employees, he succeeded in hav-

4 This integration speaks to Buck's comments about cure.

5 Gütersloh is a city in North Rhine-Westphalia and home to a well-known asylum.

> ing an almost 100% occupation rate of his residents. He achieved improvements and positive changes in pathologies that had until then been thought impossible. He proved that many problems previously only attributed to the course of the pathology in fact had more to do with environment and milieu. Sedatives could be spared and wards that had previously been locked could be opened. The successes of the Simon System were looked on everywhere as revolutionary; attempts to introduce it in other institutions failed for the most part. The Simon successes couldn't be achieved in the least elsewhere.[6]

In 1946, Dr. Simon wasn't in Gütersloh anymore. There was little to be seen of his "immense effort"; in the meantime, the institution ran, and its methods were taken for granted. The nurses seemed to me—aside from an older, somewhat stiff one—much more easygoing than in the "restless ward" in Bethel. There the work was certainly much harder because we were just being kept without any occupation and had no choice but to become restless; the nurses had to deal with that, and they seemed to me accordingly stressed and unhappy. In Gütersloh, the ward atmosphere was less stressed; it seemed cheerful and full of resolve. The number of patients were about three times that in Bethel but in percentages fewer nurses were needed. The composition of patients was about the same as in the "restless ward" in Bethel.

The institutions of the Inner Mission did not attempt to enact an "almost 100% occupation rate" of their patients, as discussed in the textbook. The Institution pastors and doctors who came together in Treysa in 1931 probably

6 Kasper Jaspersen, *Lehrbuch der Geistes- und Nervenkrankenpflege* (Bethel bei Bielefeld: Verlagshandlung der Anstalt Bethel, 1965). Simon was a German psychiatrist who stressed active treatments and holistic care, a record tarnished as he later leaned toward national socialism.

didn't know about the Gütersloh experiments, although the work therapy model had been enacted for eight years by then. Otherwise, the Institution could hardly have decided that patients whose "full occupational possibility would in all likelihood not be regained" would receive "services of care" only, within the realm of "humane care and safekeeping." That in Bethel no one knew about the successes in Gütersloh, only twenty kilometers away, was clear even in 1939, during the euthanasia actions. During these actions, occupational potential and performance decided the life and death of patients. Looking back at the euthanasia period, the Bethel information newsletter *Der Ring* (*The Ring*) of October 1983, reads:

> In fact, the question of occupational potential was of utmost importance. According to the general opinion back then it was assumed that the 'institutionalized' usually weren't capable of working. That is why Bethel made a point of classifying as many patients as possible as capable of working. That way one hoped in Bethel to get the majority of patients out of the danger zone so that in a worst case scenario there would only be as small a group as possible for which one would have to fight.[7]

It would have been more appropriate not just to classify patients on paper as "able to work" but to have actually given them opportunities to work. If Hermann Simon's work therapy had established itself in all institutions, it would have been impossible to talk about "useless

7 During the Aktion T4 period, life and death were determined on the basis of questionnaires filled out by medical personnel and graded with pluses and minuses at a headquarters in Berlin. Generally those who could be shown capable of meaningful work were spared. Bethel does not seem to have had moral problems with sterilization.

eaters."[8] The logic of the murder action, the prerequisite for removing any moral scruples, would have been robbed of justification. The director of the notorious gassing institution Hadamar, Dr. Gorgaß,[9] apparently tried to save patients from "euthanasia" through work therapy. In her report *The Killing of the Mentally Ill in Germany,* Alice Platen-Hallermund writes: "He also tried to make an inroad with Brack[10] to introduce work therapy and thus save patients from being gassed; but Brack refused all of his suggestions."[11] Now it was too late.

The active life in the Gütersloh institution impressed me. I didn't see any patients lying around in bed or sitting in resignation. The daily rhythm kept us busy. Cardiazol and insulin shocks were not used in our ward. Sleeping pills were the only medication we were given and even these were only provided at night if requested. There was no paralyzing paraldehyde. Only a very agitated young girl received sedative injections. She had fallen in love with an occupying British soldier. She died after a few days. She was rolled out of her single room through the large group hall. There she lay as if she were sleeping. A very beautiful girl.

Our ward was overfilled back then. A day room with wooden benches and long tables. On the wall a framed colorful print, in front of the windows flowerpots. Next to it a large sleeping hall with a few smaller rooms and upstairs an eight-bed room, finally the bathroom and the dressing room, where our personal clothing was kept. We only wore it on Sundays. During the week we wore

8 "Nutzloser Esser," the Nazi term for those who were disabled or medically unfit to contribute economically. These were targeted for death.

9 Hans Bodo Gorgaß did in fact gas thousands of patients at Hadamar and was sentenced to life imprisonment.

10 Viktor Brack was a Nazi and one of the architects of T4.

11 Alice Platen-Hallermund, *Die Tötung Geisteskranker in Deutschland* (Frankfurt am Main: Verlag der Frankfurter Hefte, 1948), 100.

dark blue work frocks with thin white stripes and strange white cloth trousers that were bound over rough long cloth shirts.

Following a meager breakfast—in 1946 there wasn't much to eat yet—the work groups spread out. Kitchen work was especially popular since there were always some scraps one might get. We were glad to get out of the locked ward this way. As a "newly admitted" patient I had to stay in that ward in the beginning. In the dayroom we turned old envelopes inside out and glued them again—paper was also in short supply. If one of us got restless doing this, others would tell us that everyone who became restless or even rebellious would be punished with a "vomit injection" after which one would be totally nauseated. Luckily that was over.

Later I belonged to the ironing brigade. After the midday meal we took a seated break. Then we started to work again till five or four-thirty. Nowadays, where there are steam presses and potato peeling machines, the patients in Gütersloh have more economical and especially more creative work; they get a share of the profits. Professor Klaus Dörner[12] is following new paths as director, providing employment and housing so that long-term patients can be discharged into a self-directed life.

Manfred Bleuler, an earlier director of the renowned "Burghölzli" in Zurich, had suggested toy production that leaves room for the imagination. I liked that idea a lot. There was little imagination to be found in Gütersloh back then; Prussian authoritarian order ruled. A few original characters among the patients, who had been there a long time, made comments about it with irony-filled ease. At any rate, we liked our ward nurse who was real and upbeat, and also another nurse who was very warm-hearted.

12 Klaus Dörner was a pioneer of social, community-based psychiatric care.

We got lunch in rows of two, each pair with a pot with a handle between us. In one pot with a handle there was a little bit of meat back then — for the nurses' room. In another one dessert — also for the nurses. Once, even some little strawberries. We sniffed when nobody was looking. The daily fee was five Reichsmark (RM), which was one-hundred-and-fifty RM a month. I still remember that because I paid the four-hundred-and-fifty RM for three months from my part of my brother's bequest; at the end of my service obligation my health insurance membership ran out and I'd failed to get insurance voluntarily. One could live pretty well on one-hundred-and-fifty RM a month even without being in the institution back then.

Saturday evenings the big moment arrived when our own clothing was laid out for Sunday. An older patient managed the clothes room. She took her post very seriously. Otherwise, patients were given no responsibility for managing their own things. The change from institutional garb to our own clothing was really a highlight in the monotonous day-to-day of a closed ward. Sunday itself was bleak. In the morning we went to a service — also to get out of the locked ward. The rest of the day we sat in the dayroom and played Sorry! or Chinese checkers. Those were the only two games there were. We were only allowed to go into the garden, which was separated by a low chain-link fence and a hedge, in accompaniment of a nurse. That had been the same in Frankfurt; in Bethel we'd been allowed to go into the garden alone and I liked that much better. That way we could be there much more often and for longer periods of time.

Every fourth Sunday there was a regular institution party in the afternoon. I experienced three of these parties: a dance party with a big fire department band or some other association with similar uniforms, a soccer tournament, and one afternoon on a large party lawn with games and prizes. Even today I think with joy about how someone wanted to give us these opportunities. That's how modest an institution patient becomes, knowing they belong to the lowest group in the hierarchy.

For long-term patients, this authoritarian-run mass system would have been much harder to bear than it was for me. Because I knew from the start that, as with my two previous stays, my time would be limited to two or three months. During our weekly bath, as an example of this system, the next person to bathe had to stand at the ready, undressed behind the tub, so as not to waste time with breaks. It was like being on an assembly line: let the water drain, draw a new bath, next person please! For me it was interesting as a live model subject; my fellow female patients would have found standing at the ready behind the tub more as something degrading. My mother wouldn't have been able to imagine me as a patient here.

My younger sister visited me and brought me a tablet weaver that she set up for me. Since we were fully occupied every workday, I didn't try out weaving braids. It seemed complicated with all those threads that could easily get tangled. When relatives provide occupation where there is none, it can be very helpful. I preferred to talk to the other female patients after work and on Sundays. In contrast to the "restless ward" in Bethel, we were allowed to talk to one another.

The institution director visited the wards weekly and greeted the patients. It is customary in communal institutions with medical directors for them to do this, though not with the same regularity everywhere. The head nurse came more frequently, probably daily.

During these three months, I had a dream that depressed me for days. So the ward doctor, a man who I felt had a wordless connection with us, convinced me to try electroshocks.[13] Luckily, I only received three, because

13 Electroshock causes a grand mal seizure. Without a paralytic drug it can cause not only damage to the tongue but broken bones.

during the third I bit deeply into my tongue during the spasm. I almost completely forgot the dream after that—at least it didn't depress me anymore. But then it wasn't just the dream I forgot. The effect of the spasm and the shock treatments rely on forgetting. In the process of remembering again, normal consciousness content slowly takes over.

The robust-natural atmosphere on the ward didn't allow for doubts. The ward doctor may not have believed the Bethel diagnosis. He told me he didn't consider my disorder to be schizophrenia, but exaggerated symptoms of puberty. "I'm too old for that." I was twenty-nine. He said age was irrelevant. It was encouraging that this ward doctor doubted the presence of a mental illness supposed to be incurable. But during the start of my first break in 1936, I experienced the transition from the normal stresses of puberty to psychosis, with its epiphanies and transformed experience of the world, and I knew the difference. Even the difficult states of agitation and confusion in the "restless ward" in Bethel were still present in my memory. Certainly, the complete isolation and the inhumane treatment surrounded by Bible quotes would have even confused a healthy person. But they wouldn't have experienced the shared level of symbols with which I was wordlessly connected with the other female patients.[14]

The Gütersloh institution did not let us locked-up patients have anything of our own back then, including responsibility for ourselves or self-initiative. The significance of having these, even today, means it isn't necessary to have unoccupied patients just being safeguarded. That this situation still exists in closed wards and communal and parochial houses, that the initiative

Memory loss is a common side effect.

14 The common symbolic reality of psychosis is further developed in Buck's letters.

of locked-up patients is paralyzed by psychotropic drugs, worries me deeply. I know from my own experience what it means to be forced to do nothing and to simply be held. Apparently, the responsible institution directors and doctors can't imagine what that's like. And perhaps they don't know anymore that as early as 1923, Hermann Simon introduced an "almost 100% occupation rate" and achieved this without medication.

For a long time, I didn't think Gütersloh had fed anyone into the "euthanasia" program — all the patients worked. I'd read in 1960 in *Medicine without Humanity* "that according to Conti's instructions [doctor and SS group leader and Reich health director] in the data sheet for the questionnaire, Number I, all patients who can be positively occupied in institutional facilities do not fall under the mandate to report and accordingly, the only criterion [for death] was the ability to work and nothing else."[15] However, that was an error. The West German Broadcasting's "Critical Diary"[16] said on August 17, 1983: "Of the 1022 total deported patients from Gütersloh, of which about one hundred survived, about two-thirds were deported after the supposed cessation of the extermination program."

Incomprehensible that contrary to the guidelines of the data sheet for the question form, so many working patients from one single institution were sent off to be killed.

"Dr. J. [the chief physician of our Bethel house] started the initiative from Bethel to inform all institution directors of Westphalian sanatoria, and called on them to

15 Alexander Mitscherlich and Fred Mielke, eds., *Medizin ohne Menschlichkeit: Dokumente des Nürnberger Ärzteprozesses* (Frankfurt: Fischer, 1960).

16 "Kritisches Tagebuch" ("Critical Diary") was a weekday radio show on the Westdeutsche Rundfunk (WDR, West German Broadcasting), running from 1967 to 2003.

refuse to fill out the forms,"[17] our female assistant doctor in Bethel wrote in a letter to the editor in the May 17, 1961 issue of the *Spiegel*. The institution director in Gütersloh — it wasn't the same one I experienced — had also been informed. So, he had to have known that the deported patients were going to be killed.

Before I read this shocking news, I had the impression that I'd had incomparably better experiences in Gütersloh in 1946 than the reporters Uwe Heitkamp and Michael Herl did in a number of institutions across West Germany forty years later. I did not experience in Gütersloh the complete suppression system they talked about in 1986, with belts around the abdomen, plus hand and foot restraints. In the other houses as well, there can't have been restraining measures since everyone was working.

Today — since 1984 — Klaus Dörner in Gütersloh leads the fight with support from many others, especially members of the German Society for Humanistic Psychiatry, for recognition of those killed by "euthanasia" and those forcibly sterilized as victims of the Nazi state. That this initiative should arise from psychiatry itself after fifty years, considering that its dogma of genetically determined "endogenous" psychosis created the prerequisites for the extermination efforts, I find very encouraging.

17 Letter from Dr. Med. Gertrud Runge in the section "Briefe," *Spiegel*, May 16, 1961, https://www.spiegel.de/politik/sterbehilfe-a-4b52ac67-0002-0001-0000-000043364022. Buck erroneously dates the issue to May 17.

8

The Stone Blossom

After three months I was discharged. My mother picked me up and took me to a single room in the neurological ward of an open house at Bethel for a month. It was situated across from the closed house I had been in in 1936. A Bethel pastor who was friends with my parents had offered them that. From here I was supposed to look for a room in Bielefeld in order to continue my education, which had been interrupted by the closure of the academies, at the vocational art school there.

I'd never wanted to return to Bethel again. But I also had doubts about the professor in Bielefeld after having visited him with Mother. Our instructor in Frankfurt, with his admiration for early Greek sculpture, the intensity of his own work, and his spontaneous reactions to ours, conveyed a sense of form that fed itself from within, through its tension and interaction with the senses. After working with this man and teacher, going to another whose formal language leaned toward the decorative wasn't going to be easy. It was hard to find a room in 1946, but I also didn't put much effort into it and never found one.

From my window I looked out at the closed house with the "restless ward" where I'd experienced the most oppressive events of my life. Painful memories of the forcible sterilization rose in me again. The same doctors also ran the neurological ward that was adjacent to a nursing home.

This wasn't the right place; what my parents had found for me was not my path. This feeling probably favored an after-break. And my psychosis was also probably not completely in remission. Otherwise, the following wouldn't have been possible.

Among the female patients on the ward there was a young deacon who experienced multiple attacks daily. She lost consciousness for brief periods and then was prone to injure herself. I witnessed one of these attacks as we were sitting outside in a large circle shelling peas or something like that. At that moment I was overcome by the certainty that this would be her last attack. I went up to her room with her right after it happened. She still seemed spaced out. I told her she was now done with attacks and wrote on a little card that Jesus has cured her. I was so certain of her cure that I explained to her she wouldn't need any more medication and poured her medicine out of the window. Now we took long walks together; she hadn't had the confidence to do that previously. And in fact, she did not have any subsequent episodes. Soon after, she was discharged. Such certainties only overcame me when I was in a psychotic state.

At the end of these four weeks, I was deeply moved by the press photo of the former lawyer Robert Kempner, who had been denaturalized by Hitler and helped prepare the international military tribunal in Nuremberg from 1942 on. He now represented the prosecution. Kempner was laughing in the photo. Everyone was waiting for the death sentences. The accused who had themselves brought so much death and misery to millions of human beings now had to accept their sentences, but Kempner's laughing appalled me. I felt that the prosecutors had no reason to show arrogance. The destruction of our cities under whose rubble a helpless civilian population had died, and the atom bombs dropped on Hiroshima and

Nagasaki were also war crimes. Kempner's laughter perhaps had nothing to do with the death sentences; perhaps the photojournalist just happened to get him in front of the camera as he laughed about some banal matter. But I automatically saw the laughter in context to his function as an American prosecutor. Here in Bethel where all the old wounds were opening again, my sensitivity was especially elevated.

I was so outraged by the prosecutor's laughter that I created an ad in the Bielefeld newspaper in which I invited the city to the main square for a meeting. I named the topic "The true guilty of the First and Second World War." I named my former colleague from drawing class at the Frankfurt Art Academy as the speaker; his name seemed to have more drawing power than mine as a woman. And since an ad by an occupant of Bethel would hardly have been published, I used the address of the street that goes from Bethel to Bielefeld and as a house number a random one that occurred to me. I later realized that this exact number was missing on that street. As far as I know, the ad was published, though I had no doubt that people would be protesting the war crimes of the allied forces at this meeting.

The following night, I was picked up from bed and taken to the doctors' room by the female chief physician — our assistant doctor from 1936. There were Englishmen in uniform sitting there. They wanted to know who the truly guilty were. I was better at speaking English than at any other time in my life and I explained that through the edict of Versailles they had created the conditions for Hitler's rise and thus were also guilty for his war. A not quite convincing course of reasoning. But some of my most vivid childhood memories concerned the millions in war debt that Germany had to come up with following the Versailles treaty[1]; on my way to the baker's, I read the debt numbers in big white lettering on a long red brick garden wall, and daily so many beggars came. I connected their visits with this gigantic debt. Following the conversation, I was taken to the closed house opposite on the very same night and thus apparently dodged an arrest.

Today, as I report on my institution experiences, I almost feel grateful for my renewed admission. And Bethel probably, too. Because without it, my primarily negative impressions of Bethel would have remained unchanged. Much had changed since 1936. Now there was even an admission protocol: a young female assistant doctor in a white coat sat in front of me and typed into a typewriter what I told her. It still wasn't an actual conversation. I was not asked what had led me to place this ad. No one was interested, because common wisdom still held that psychoses had physical determinants and were subsequently meaningless.

Because I was embarrassed to have been admitted back, I claimed an angel at home advised me to have myself admitted for this second time. And she typed the angel into her machine without asking further questions. There was a kernel of truth in the angel story, in that Molt's face in a dream led me to leave home.

I was put in the half open ward, in which a regular group of long-term patients lived with the same number of transition patients in comfortable single and double bedrooms, occupied with house and garden work, sewing and mending and running errands. With the two nice nurses who were also responsible for the lab we formed a ward community. At the end of the long hallways with the bedrooms and a tea kitchen was the living room, at the other end the sewing room.

1 After this post-World War I 1919 treaty, Germany entered a desperate period of hyperinflation.

The lovingly tended garden with its roofed pergola was overgrown with climbing plants. These covered the walls on the broad side and encouraged lively contact between the patients of three wards. Only the patients from the "restless" and the "quiet" wards were excluded from this community; they had their own gardens that were surrounded by high walls. I don't like this exclusion. The more contacts the sicker patient has with the healthier the more favorable it is for them. Maybe keeping the healthier ones apart from the sicker is appropriate around the very young. Schizophrenic patients have a lot of understanding for one another because they share similar experiences; group conversations could deepen this understanding.

Fellow female patients told me that the "restless" ward was now being run by a loving, cheerful nurse and thus almost sought after by some. That was good to know because the atmosphere of an institution depends on how the sickest patients are treated. Of course, we shared these kinds of experiences with one another.

The nurses lived in the house; it was their home. This gave it a domestic character. They ate lunch and dinner with the patients of the open and partially open ward; a few female patients from the ward for the depressed also joined us. There was the same food for everyone, not like in Gütersloh where the better food was for the nurses and the worse for the patients. After meals, the house mother read something aloud out of a book, like the *Memories of Youth of an Old Man* by Wilhelm von Kügelgen.[2] Even such small things can take the monotony out of institutional life.

There was also some land that belonged to the house. "We are now going to harvest the last bit before the frost comes," I wrote my parents, "gigantic kohlrabi, red beets,

2 Wilhelm von Kügelgen, *Jugenderinnerungen eines alten Mannes* (Ebenhausen bei München: W. Langewiesche-Brandt, 1922).

the last tomatoes, the fruit is down but the vegetable garden still looks colorful with endive, red, green, and white cabbage, leeks, etc. Garden and farm work make me very happy."

I was responsible for daily sweeping of the dining room with its horseshoe of tables, mopping and polishing and setting the tables for meals; I was supposed to set up chairs for Bible studies and I accompanied the chorales at the piano. I was also responsible for the library and in the first weeks I discovered *The Year of the Lord* by Karl Heinrich Waggerl.[3] The Austrian poet describes the farm life of a mountain village with its Catholic feast days in this novel.

The lively, earthly piety of this book drew me in, especially then in Bethel. Because there was no space for the world with its joys in this "City of God." Unlike Gütersloh, there were no diversions like dance or soccer here; girls were also not allowed to dance together. Every figure in this book is drawn in understanding and loving detail. The old village pastor who tends to his garden and field himself doesn't walk around with Bible quotes in his mouth when he visits the sick Monika. Instead hidden in each of his hands there's an apple: "Right or left?" Most of all I was enchanted by little David, Monika's son, who grows up alone in the village poorhouse, while his mother lives far away in the city. He always thinks of something, or something happens to him, to fill his impoverished life with adventure.

In a letter to my parents, I find the effect of this book and its author mirrored onto myself. And I also find the strong self-confidence I had with all my breaks. I also find myself a little crazy in this letter: not in the later ones. Very slowly, my psychosis subsided without medication this time; the strong impulses of the acute break reverted

3 Karl Heinrich Waggerl, *Das Jahr des Herrn* (Wiesbaden: Insel-Verlag, 1933).

bit by bit into a now just-weak instinct. That was an important experience for me; following the medication-induced interruption of the previous breaks in Ilten and Frankfurt I hadn't experienced that. Now I learned that the strong impulses which I felt as "guidance," and in the first break experienced as the "driving spirit" according to Paul, all were drawn from an instinct that actually came out of me. The psychiatrist usually isn't aware of how important it is for the patient to understand this context. The schizophrenic experiences the inner impulse — or the inner voice, everyone calls it something else — first as a strong driving force that they think is coming from the outside as some sort of "epiphany."

It was the beginning of December, so shortly before Christmas, when I wrote the letter:

> Dear parents! Here is my wish list for Christmas, I'd love to have these things as soon as possible because we need them for our plans. And they are all just *my* things that I'd like you to send, because I don't want anything else. Actually, Miss A. and I would like to make a fairytale book together: the fairytales by me, the design by Miss. A. And to do that we need a lot of my beautiful white-and-yellow paper from the rolls, not the Ingres sheets. Additionally, some of my water-color paints, the ones in the box that says "materials," perhaps three from all of the color cups. Then some sturdy cardboard as well. Then for the banners that Miss A. wants to draw, some of my transparent paper. You must just see what you find. Miss A. needs to be immersed in her work in order to make progress.
>
> Then, for my little friend Lieselotte, the case that occupies me the most here, my recorder series of music notes and, should we have some, easy piano music — that too. I am now working on notes she didn't know yet (she is thirteen), and the very simple things on the piano, and I have experienced miracles through

> the child by steering her away from the intensity of her illness to something that interests her very much. Previously I only got to hear about her back pain, heavy feet, intestinal worms, etc. Now all of that has receded into the background. "You've made me healthy, not at all the doctors," she said this morning. But she's not quite that far along yet.
>
> Actually, except with Karl Heinrich Waggerl, I don't spend anywhere near as much time with any person as with her, strange somehow. I was never able to talk to anyone like this except of course with Karl Heinrich. We have almost identical sensations—that makes me very happy. Should I at some point earn enough money, which I am sure about, I will take over her whole musical education because it surprises me how strong her feeling is for the beauty in melodies. She works with great intensity and that is why I believe she will get somewhere with music. This seriousness about the piano will never leave her because she *needs* the music due to her inherited depression. It's something different from the person who chooses music due to talent. And the talent will grow in her. Her voice is also very beautiful.

My parents are sure to have worried about my conversation with Karl Heinrich Waggerl, but of course I was only talking to him in my thoughts. When you imagine the situation of a person who is isolated from the outside world—I did not have permission to leave the premises—then such conversations with a far-removed stranger sound less strange. The unrealistic assessment of my financial future must also have worried my parents; at least I felt sure I would at some point be able to take over expenses for Lieselotte's music education.

Miss A., with whom I wanted to make the fairytale book, belonged to the long-term patients. She suffered from an enlarged thyroid; years later she had an operation from which she died. Her parents had had a farm in the East; she'd tended the smaller animals and the garden. She wasn't able to get over the loss of her native farm and circle of friends; she was often despondent. Her father visited her fairly frequently.

I stayed in the Bethel house for one-and-three-quarter years, and it became dear to me because this time the good sides outweighed the bad. Soon I was allowed to sculpt after cleaning up the dining room following breakfast. From the profit of my fired ceramics, I could now pay for my stay myself (at a very reduced price). I found friends among my fellow patients and nursed and befriended the family of the chief physician. Some discharged patients stayed in touch with the house for years by letter.

After Lieselotte, I shared the room with Sister H., a deaconess. She explained her presence was due to an incurable vascular constriction from which she suffered. She didn't tell me anything further about the effects, but she lived in constant fear of this illness. One night, I experienced what it was that she was afraid of. She transitioned into a deep psychotic state as if coming from a dream, or still caught in one. The strangest thing for me was that she spoke a different language. She emphasized the second syllable of each word, instead of the first, as was common in German. The language sounded French, but the words indicated clearly that it wasn't. As a student in a public elementary school this patient hadn't learned French; she also couldn't have heard it from her parents who had themselves only been to the public school –Volksschule went to ninth grade. But I knew that she came from a family of Huguenots. By her looks — she was petite and dark — she could have been French. Had an inherited, old speaking rhythm broken out in her psychosis?

Sister H. became very restless. She apparently was afraid of snake hallucinations. I called the ward nurse, but she couldn't calm her down either. Sister H. was taken to the "restless" ward, which was perhaps not so restless anymore. Upon returning after weeks, she didn't want to say anything further about her psychosis experiences. She only said that they had been terrible. Among the many female patients I met over the course of my time in institutions, Sister H. was one of the few who had only suffered from her psychotic experiences. I got the impression that it was exactly her fear of an unalterable fate that made her experiences so torturous and frightening. Through her I experienced vividly how disastrous it is for the patient to believe that psychosis is an incurable physiological illness. The vascular constriction which she thought she suffered from, and which she was afraid of, was perhaps simply her personal image for this incurable and incomprehensible process which, according to doctors, expressed itself in the body of the psychotic person. She felt punished by God with an incurable suffering. Had she been able to understand her psychosis as a mental issue, as something that she could influence through her trust in God, then she would have probably also experienced the positive sides of her unconscious.

We still find schizophrenia explained in dictionaries today as having a physiological cause and thus being incurable.

There are probably few patients for whom their psychiatric sentence doesn't become the heaviest burden in their lives. I was helped a little by having consciously experienced the development of my first break over the course of five weeks, recognizing the connection of the psychotic context with the preceding mental conflict. The diagnosis still hit me lethally, and new breaks had to constantly liberate me from the feeling that I was not a whole human being as a "mentally ill woman." I didn't know yet that the source of my psychosis lay in my own unconscious. I also didn't know that it is a quality of the unconscious to break into consciousness forcefully and to lead to changes in the normal thinking process which we call an "epiphany."

This understanding didn't become clear to me until my fifth break, which was then able to be my last one. The encounter with Sister H. was an important step in getting there. The foreign language that she spoke during her psychotic break, and which sounded so markedly similar to the language of her Huguenot ancestors, made me think for the first time that everyone must have their own subconscious storing very old experiences, and these break open in psychosis. But I still knew too little about the idiosyncrasies and abilities of this unconscious to refer to my psychotic experiences correctly as epiphanies, and not as something else. As long as I felt they had been epiphanies (given from without) I simply considered them reality and trusted them, without making it clear to myself that they had to be understood symbolically.

In spite of her fears, Sister H. had not felt completely deserted. "He carried everything with me. He knew about everything," she told me when she returned from the "restless" ward. She was referring to the chief physician.

I understood how she could have this feeling about him. His conversations didn't need conscious understanding; he seemed to live from a broad human perspective, so Sister H. could feel accepted and understood though he knew little about her experience. He and the Gütersloh ward doctor, among the twenty institutional doctors, professors, and assistant doctors I experienced, were the only ones who had a nonverbal contact with their patients and perhaps they didn't even know they did. "We don't know anything," this chief physician once told me. This honesty also made him trustworthy. Other institution doctors gave themselves the air of being so knowledgeable and self-assured.

None of these doctors was capable of explaining things. Not even here. One didn't speak about our psychosis here either. I can think of one single short conversation with the female chief physician. We were in the garden; I mentioned the heightened sensitivity during psychosis. "Other patients have told me that already, that it's as if one only had a very thin skin," she said. But that was it. No one mentioned the forcible sterilization and its effects.

But we were respected as human beings. What the individual contributed to the familial community of the house was more important than their "illness." Of course, there were also difficulties. In one of my letters to my parents I wrote: "And it's no wonder that the people with their confusing life situations sap one's energy, one can't help—when one tries, one is put in one's place as a patient and external possibilities of helping are taken away. You must try to think your way into this difficult situation."

The doctor suggested that as of August 1 I should go to Worpswede for six weeks to get a change of air. "He couldn't have said to me anything more wonderful," I wrote my parents:

> I can finance this now.... My work slump is already over and since there is a ceramicist in Worpswede I want to try to make the two nativities for O. there so that I get done with my orders. That I can be here again afterwards, especially for the winter, makes me very happy because this house really seems more and more like the right place for me. I can hardly imagine a life in a small community like, a family, maybe just because only one part of me gets motivated there, whereas in a living community with lots of facets and many different types of people, as is the case here, there are many more connections.

At first, I hadn't wanted to be in Bethel at all and now I had acclimated very well. But was it just about Bethel? The letter continues:

> I often think about the constant need to reduce oneself as one reason for my illness, because every time prior to the breaks there was an effort to converse or to share my thoughts etc., even the last time. But nobody ever answered. Now I don't expect a break because my inner space has grown and somehow, without many words, there are counter-balancing poles there. Tensions and explosions can't develop at all anymore in that exaggerated form. And I really owe this to this house.

With the "nobody answered," I suppose I meant the lack of conversations, the need to exclude what happened in my psychosis, with the "constant need to reduce oneself" to meet the permitted norms. That is why Waggerl's Little David became so important to me with his imaginative transformations and reinterpretation of reality. His author could only have made him up drawing on the experiences of his own childhood. But the conversations with my fellow female patients also gave me a lot. Especially those I had with a long-term female patient in our ward, whom I found especially endearing—she stands out vividly with her "free associations," whose meaning I could only imagine.

A hierarchical order—at the top the doctors as academics, under them the nurses and care providers, and at the very bottom the patients—did not exist here because the house belonged to the nursing staff. Our house mother, whom I'd met in 1936 as the oldest nurse in the house, was surely twenty years older than the chief physician. Both were strong personalities with natural authority, and they had great mutual respect. Only a few years had passed since the end of the wild euthanasia, the common work on behalf of threatened patients, the day-and-night-long rewording of all patient records for long-term patients, the removal of especially threatened ones to family or private care, created a close connection between doctors and nurses.

Our chief physician had been suspicious as soon as the application forms[4] arrived in June or July of 1940 and tried to get to the bottom of things with Pastor Fritz von Bodelschwingh.[5] When he saw his suspicion confirmed, he brought a charge of murder to the Stapo (state police) office in Bielefeld and with the Gestapo in Berlin. He informed the directors and doctors of other institutions about the forms, and also told leading clerics and the physicians' chamber.[6] He tried to convince them to agree on a rejection of "euthanasia" and on communal resistance to collecting patient information on the forms. Through him Bishop von Galen found out about the "euthanasia" murders at the end of July 1940. But I only heard about this many years later.

Here it became clear to me that a humane psychiatric ward started with the architectural plan. By making the dining room the center of the house and having a common garden, one created the conditions for a house community. Without the two closed wards for "restless" and "quiet" female patients, who were excluded from the community—even their gardens were separated by a high wall from the common garden—this two-story house could have been the model for a smaller psychiatric clinic that could work in any city. The covered pergola could have glass doors, be heated in winter, and have work rooms for musical and other occupations; the patients would then be able to see the garden and would feel less locked up. I find it much worse than walls to be allowed out of the building only accompanied, and only during specific times, to get fresh air. With the current

4 Buck is referring to the list of questions determining life or death under T4.

5 The pastor supported sterilization, but not death.

6 It's important to note about Aktion T4 that some doctors refused to participate, with few or no consequences.

lack of care personnel sometimes this means not getting out for days or even weeks at a time.

One develops through one's actions. The more these involve the whole person, the less space there is for troubling mental experiences. It seems to me an important task for the psychiatric ward to let patients figure out what kind of offerings of education, arts, and crafts are satisfying and fulfilling for them. Discharged ward patients are often unemployed or go into retirement early; they must develop the ability to live meaningful lives on a daily basis. To do that they must figure out where their interests and gifts lie. Living and working spaces should be separated from one another just as in normal life. Even patients in a closed ward, for whom daily meaningful occupation is especially important as a support, should be able to go into the garden alone.

The thirteen-year-old Lieselotte overcame her ailment by diverting her interest from the ailment to learning how to play the piano. I had the same experience following the forcible sterilization. Initially, it was only the thought of having the freedom to commit suicide that kept me going. But once I began with pottery, using the wheel, and found the possibility of expressing myself through sculpting, my desperation eventually receded into the background. My work opened entirely new experiences in the expression of the forms, not just in sculpture, but also in nature. When something new comes on account of illness—the unfolding of previously untapped abilities, a new understanding of one's self through the understanding of the psychosis background—then the illness can become a positive force for the affected person. It strengthens one's self-confidence instead of weakening it, as automatically happens in the psychiatric ward without such aids—especially where even today patients are just held, put on medication, and thus forced to waste away.

Even in deeply frightening psychosis, such as Sister H.'s snake hallucinations, one can recognize a meaning. Only if one cannot recognize their symbolic meaning can psychotic images seem scary. "A snake is coming out of my mouth," a schizophrenic female patient said. In Ernst Kretschmer's *Medical Psychology* I read: "Northwest American Indigenous People represented the soul as it fled the body with a human figure sitting on a birdlike ship and from its mouth a snake was emerging."[7] The snake is a symbol of vital force that leaves the human being in death. The shedding snake is a symbol of renewal. The bird that evolved from the reptile-like awareness in the subconscious is not, like the snake, bound to the earth — the body — and thus can represent the soul fleeing the body, here as a birdlike ship on its way to another world, which comes after earthly life. The snake leaving the body — "a snake is coming out of my mouth" — can also mean the death of the old person, which precedes renewal and rebirth, and thus becomes a symbol of development. In my case this symbolic death prior to rebirth didn't express itself as a fleeing snake but as the sinking in the mudflats.

Worpswede didn't work out; I couldn't find lodging. In the winter I drew a lot on the blackboard I had received from another patient. "This way I can save my paper while I'm drawing," I wrote home, "and one works more freely it seems if one can wipe it off right away." We were all sitting in the dining room close to the stove because it was bitter cold.

But then there was a new plan: for four to six weeks I'd go to Munich for live-model drawing. If I could find lodging there. And definitely before the devaluation of the currency which was now expected to come in June of 1948. The end of April 1948 I got on a train to Munich. The

7 Ernst Kretschmer, *Medizinische Psychologie*, 3rd ed. (Leipzig: Georg Thieme, 1926), 68.

ward nurse and another nurse came to the railway station to say goodbye and brought along sandwiches, candy, and cookies for me.

"So here I am in Munich after a 24-hour ride, which was nonetheless pleasant," I wrote my parents:

> Munich seems pretty depressing and totally changed. Additionally, incredibly expensive [...]. And on top of that the Academy is only partially operational, the drawing classes are all still in Dachau. And so I will go to the mountains early tomorrow morning and go hiking. That will give me more than this depressing city. Perhaps I can draw on the way.

Nine days later I was already writing from Salzburg:

> I've been in Austria since the 3rd and have drawn a lot. I'm really getting back into it and am very happy about it. There are four of us: two young women from Wolfenbüttel and one from Hamburg but born in Vienna. We have a wonderful fellowship and share everything with each other. I hope very much that I may stay in Austria until after Pentecost, which nowadays is so difficult. I like this country and its people so much. From here I want to first go to Berchtesgaden and Königsee and then to Munich [...]. All four of us dodged the fare crossing the border, me automatically, without knowing we had already crossed over onto Austrian ground.

That I was writing from jail, where we were locked up for ten days, I thought better not to mention to my parents. We'd been taken in for "unpermitted border crossing." The policeman who checked our IDs was tactful enough to show me a few Salzburg sites on the way to jail.

The end of May I had to return to Munich to see a dentist because of a root canal. I also went to the Academy that had been severely damaged by bombs. Our Frankfurt professor had been called to the Munich Academy after the war; but I didn't see him, he had taken off on travels. "One can't work all that well," I wrote home, "the nutrition is probably too bad. In the other classes work was even worse. And so I'm thinking of moving to drawing in the next months and to progress enough to get contracts for portraits."

I saw paintings from the destroyed Pinakothek in the Haus der Kunst, an exhibition of sculptures by Marcks, Maillol, and Lehmbruck,[8] and a Paul Klee exhibition in the house of a sculptor. And then I was back in the mountains. I wrote to my parents from the Rossfeld Hut:

> I am just getting back from Austria where I had a wonderful weekend and was fed very well [...]. Without any incidents, I made it here from the hut and back. The first truck with its new liquid manure trailer that I flagged down was headed to Wagrain where the author Heinrich Waggerl lived. I ran into him by complete chance on the village street and since I love his book *The Year of the Lord* we struck up a conversation right away. I actually now wanted to head to St. Johann but he thought I should better stay in Wagrain, which was of course my preference too [...]. A film director and an actress from the Vienna Burg Theater, who had made a film in which she played the lead, were also there, and in the evening we met at Waggerl's for a cozy gathering.

Of course, it wasn't by "complete chance" that I met Waggerl. In my knapsack, besides a bag of oats and a glass of marmalade, I also had a stone blossom I wanted to bring him; I had found it in the plaza in front of the cathedral of Mainz among the rubble. And the encounter had not

8 Artists Gerhard Marcks, Aristide Maillol, and Wilhelm Lembruck.

occurred completely without obstacles. I stood in front of the house in which Waggerl lived and saw behind the window a man sitting at a typewriter. No, I didn't just see him, I could also hear him. Apparently, he read what he had just typed, the same way I do. Something vain seemed to swing in his voice. I turned around deeply disappointed. I had gone to such effort to meet Waggerl and his mountain village. I had taken the train to St. Johann from Salzburg. But it hadn't been the right St. Johann. The train conductor explained that Wagrain was close to St. Johann in Pongau. I had to walk a long way back to Salzburg. As it was getting dark, I found a little cave a bit to the side of the street I could just fit into to sleep. In the morning a big spider crawled out from under the stone I had used as a pillow. Not a good sign, I thought. And then there was the ID check at the Salzburg train station and my arrest. My feet were sore but could heal well in jail, and we didn't need to give up our food stamps in order to be fed.

All of these adventures, and then such a disappointment! With a heavy head I returned to the village street feeling glum. A deep voice spoke to me — Karl Heinrich Waggerl stood before me. This time it was the right Waggerl. In *The Year of the Lord,* he compares every day with a stone we receive from God's hand in order to imbue it with our actions and build it into the architecture of life. That was why I had taken the little stone blossom from the ruins of war; I thought it fit well in his architecture. The fantasy of the old cathedrals seemed to have disappeared from our life. There was no more room for stone blossoms; one built with fabricated stones. But the writers kept this fantasy alive. And perhaps it still lives on in us psychotics.

On my return, Bethel gave me a sewing room in an open house to work and live in. That meant a lot back then, because after the money reform my earnings were uncertain. Since material and thread were scarce and expensive, I usually had the room to myself. The female director of the nursing home is unforgettable to me, a relatively young nurse who exuded joy even in her movements. This natural and sensitive woman also experienced depressive phases in her life; perhaps her elated joy would not have been possible without this context of heaviness. Looking back, I realize how important for different life phases are the different people who accompany them. In one's own action and feelings one switches off with the other; people, in contrast, remain unmoved in one's memory as what they were and thus can continue to have an influence. In this time, the warmhearted wife of the chief physician became very important to me, an originally talented painter. We drew portraits together of the older women in the home and she gave me good corrections. The friendly connection to the family of the chief physician made up a little for my own family, who I only visited for a few weeks around Christmas.

I drew wherever people were sitting and keeping still, in the train station waiting room, during the watchdog test, or in the Bethel plant nursery during the lunch break. There I also made some ceramic heads of a few of the workers; I also sculpted heads of many children. "I still have lots to learn until I understand forms from the inside and the outside," I wrote home. "How hard it is to work without the necessary foundation is more and more clear to me."

I actually wanted to stay in Bethel over the winter and then continue my interrupted education. But it wound up being another year and a quarter, because my parents couldn't pay to have two daughters educated simultaneously. Now the most important thing was to be financially independent. It was only possible to sell small cheap things in this time following the currency reform, and so I made thousands of candlestick holders. I pressed both my thumbs twice into a clay ball so that a flower formed around the candle hole. It went fast; it cost more energy to get the clay, and to get the many candleholders and little sculptures on a handcart to the brick factory eight kilometers away to fire and then bring them back to send them to hospitals and homes. Before Christmas, the candleholder and nativity business went well; it was more difficult to sell anything in the summer. I tried my luck with witches and monsters as piggy banks; the wide-open mouths were meant to gobble money. "I worked away at piggy banks in vain yesterday," I wrote my parents, "in the end after all the grotesque figures, another Mary appeared. But this Mary is different from the others, for the first time her form didn't come from the sense of form but from inside, a better path."

I tried to continue along this path and the chief physician's wife encouraged me. I had gotten an idea of what an internally fulfilled form could be in the last two months of the last semester, prior to the closing of the academies in 1944, but I was far away from realizing this idea. Even our professor had rarely been happy with his work. With the portrait of his wife, he found that fulfilled form in its spiritual–sensual tension, but for him it was too individual; he changed it into something more universal. This experience encouraged me to trust the immediate freshness of what came into being spontaneously.

I couldn't return to this professor when I finally continued my studies in 1950 because for the Academy, at almost thirty-three, I was too old. The universities would have taken me but they required previous vocational training. Students of the professor with whom I wanted to study recommended I do a woodworking apprenticeship in East Germany; there I was able to finish my journeyman's exam. Prior to leaving Bethel — this time filled with gratitude — I spoke with the chief physician about my psychosis, which still made me feel insecure. I wrote to my parents about this conversation: "What one really wants to say is difficult to express and what one is able to express is generally not what is essential. Dr. J.'s way of dealing with these things I liked, not so much medically but as a human being." At the end of April 1950, I left for the GDR.

The carving and wood sculpting school was located in a little mountain village. It was meant to support the cottage industry, prepare apprentices from surrounding woodworking factories for the journeyman's exam, and journeymen for the master's exam, but it also had a boarding school for those who came from far away. The remote village had stuck to its traditions. Besides Christmas, Candlemas and the Funfair[9] were the biggest village festivals. Funfair boys erected the "village linden tree," a spruce attached to a long pole with colorful ribbons and wreaths and organized the dance under this "linden tree"; simultaneously, gigantic round sheet cakes were baked in communal ovens. The border ran right along one of my landlady's lawns; it was easy to cross over it if one waited for the border policeman to pass by. Whoever was caught had to sit in jail for four days — the GDR at that time was not comparable to the later Stasi-state.

We worked well and hard in the school. Some master's students crafted life-sized nudes from beech tree trunks with such self-assurance it surprised me. There was a great willingness to offer help among the students; the feeling of community was greater than in the West. We did lots together on Sundays. I'll never forget the celebrations around the two-hundredth anniversary of Johann Sebastian Bach's death, which I experienced during summer break in the city of his birth, Eisenach. There was a wreath laying at the Bach monument, with the boys' choir singing in black ponchos and berets and many children running around; a ringing of all the church bells at the hour of his death; a nightly candlelight "Art of the Fugue" in his birth house; and the festive church service

9 The Funfair is a German public festival, with rides and activities.

that followed, with three-thousand people singing the chorale "Jesu, Joy of Man's Desiring."

Aside from practicing carving, we also worked by contract. A clock factory, for example, needed ideas for new clock cases. I worked on a mountain man out of oak for an apprentices' house and a memorial plaque for peace. There were hefty arguments around the commission of a women's league: a birthday present for Stalin that was supposed to express the connection of the German woman with "Comrade Stalin." The student body was in agreement in opposition to the teacher, who was the only representative of Stalinist communism. But the free work phase was already coming to an end. From 1952 on, figurative work was only supposed to be done by the art academy. When my journeyman's exam began at the end of January 1952, students were already forbidden to freely choose their exam piece. I was assigned the figure of a worker; size and amount of time to finish were exactly defined. Sociopolitical teaching took precedence in importance. A stricter political atmosphere was spreading.

Nonetheless, my return was not easy. The stronger sense of community that I had experienced in East Germany—wouldn't I miss it at home in West Germany?

9

The Big Chill

Ever since I came across archaic Greek sculpture in 1941, it didn't let me go. Its form seemed to come from within—creating tension, holding that form coming from inside—and with joy in its smiling faces. There isn't a standing leg and a gesture leg; these beings stand in the world on both their feet, usually with one leg in front of the other, as if the figure is headed for a goal. Like children running into the arms of their parents, they seem to be on their way to their gods. One can feel the unity of these early figures with creation itself, and with the gods. This sense of trust related to the feeling of guidance in me that came from the outbreak of instinct in my psychotic break. But would I ever be able to realize such a form, which found its tension from within?

Now I was a student at the art academy in the class of a sculptor who was dedicated to teaching. "He put a lot of value in listening to music so that we get 'momentum into our souls'," I wrote my parents. "Right now, the luck of having such a man to learn from is momentum enough. It's wonderful how his critique is individualized, for example, in drawing which is very intensive and done only with nibs." But I found the six hours a week of live model drawing too little. And during these six hours one only drew. After the last years of working figuratively from my imagination I wanted to sculpt from a natural perspective to comprehend it and thus be able to release myself from it again. Saturday afternoons, when I was alone in the class studio, I would sculpt myself as I stood in front of a big mirror. In the winter semester of 1951, I separated a corner at the back of a long hallway, which we had been relegated to because of repair work, with a curtain and could now work on a life-sized relief naked using my mirror image.

On the side, I also made works I could sell; the academy helped negotiate commissions. During the summer break I went door-to-door as a bookseller for a publishing house. The work in the group was inspiring and everyone's readiness to help was large; when I was working on the nude relief my colleagues built me a mount and set it up so I could better get to the feet. For housing I shared a room with four others in a house for female students, professionals, and apprentices close to our academy. Five in a room were actually too many, but we managed until one of us who worked in an office brought a radio home. Early morning radio, evening radio—she must have needed it to make up for her monotonous work, but I needed to prepare for the day in peace and I totally lost my rhythm. I couldn't relax anymore and couldn't sleep. I took sleeping pills because it was too difficult to find a different room back then and I didn't want to waste precious study time searching; I had to take ever more pills because I got used to them quickly and still wasn't sleeping. At home during the break, I still couldn't find sleep. I had to sit out an entire semester and also missed finishing two commissions.

Under medical supervision, I went through a sleeping pill cure; every two hours a sleeping pill, even during the day. All I did was stumble around, but I couldn't sleep. My trust in neurology experienced another crack. With hot foot baths in the evening, I finally, very slowly, found a few hours of sleep again. But I was affected for years. "You started so brilliantly and what's going on now?" our professor asked me. It took a long time for me to feel energy inside myself again.

In December of 1954, my father died; two and a half years later my mother followed him. Their entire care had been dedicated to their children and their community. Not just in words — in the years of need following the war, they had built up their own relief agency. In the spring of 1955, my professor also died. A good, experiment-happy sculptor took over the class until the position was filled again. He tried to support each student according to their specific need.

In this time — and again later — I was moved by the theme of "Mother and Child," the relationship of both, the matching up of the large and small form. In my sketches I varied the theme. Sometimes the relationship was playful, sometimes the child sheltered in its mother's encircling arms. After many smaller attempts, I finally sculpted a larger-than-life-size group. The child ventures out in its first steps out of the safety of its mother, who stands like a dark hollow behind it and leads it carefully by the hands. "That should be in a chapel," our teacher spontaneously said when he saw the sculpture for the first time. "Don't do anything else to the child!" Indeed, it looked happy, led by its mother's leading hand. That the teacher suggested this non-sacred sculpture for a sacred space was exactly what I wanted to express. I myself felt like a child being accompanied by an invisible hand.

A new professor was called to our academy in 1958 and took over the sculpting class. For the first time we again sculpted with live nude models; up to then we had only done a few weeks of nude figure drawing a week. Sculpting requires an even deeper feeling into, and understanding of, the body, and so I began to see some laws of nature, some principles I hadn't recognized drawing. It became clear to me that these laws build the foundation for free composition and creation. So after years of studying, it was only toward the end that I realized the most essential thing was still missing. We had learned to sculpt portraits from nature and to use our imagination in free works to develop our personal style. But the foundation was missing: sculpting using live nude models.

It was the academy's job to provide this foundation; it wasn't attainable just with live model drawing. Even our professors had learned to compose freely based on a comprehensive study of live models. But artists frequently let their students be where they already are; that is stimulating for both, but neglects learning the foundations. I only had a single semester left and I didn't have the means to pay a model, although I had been living off commissions for some time. How was I to make up what I had missed? The professor counseled me to request another semester. But I'd already overextended the number of semesters I could enroll in — the academy rejected my request.

It wasn't the missing live model study — the crisis went deeper, and again made me question my self-confidence. My profession was doubly important to me, because it had to replace so many other things that were unattainable since the forced sterilization: marriage, children, family. Now my studies were almost finished, and I hadn't learned the essential part. Would I ever be able to become a good sculptor now; would work still satisfy me if I kept having to realize I was missing foundations?

My deep disappointment was the trigger for my fifth break. Unsettled and with shaken self-confidence about who I was, I apparently needed the inner security I got through impulses from the unconscious. They were a little weak initially, but they again gave me the feeling of being closely woven into the whole, and difficult things seemed to succeed by themselves.

Before this last semester came to a close, I'd built a nude sculpture that was just a third of life size for a play, *The Marriage Carousel.* The actress had been my model in the theater, and I only got a few drawings. I had to have the piece done in four days. Like knitting the children's coat during the previous break, I simply let the released impulses take over my hands. The sculpture was done on time; in a normal state this would have been hard for me.

In the small, quotidian things I also experienced this sense of security in the whole. It was as if the world had a pact with me. I never had to wait for the tram as I usually did; it arrived just as I got there. There was no early or late arriving anywhere when I followed the impulses of when to head out. Even the certainty about hidden contexts began to erupt again. In this spring of 1959, summer fashion and fabrics for the first time used the color combination of green and violet. Green was the color of plants and nature, violet the union between the blue of the sky and the red of love in the Protestant church flag. In this union of green and violet I saw a sign that was the premonition of a future union developing between nature and spirit. This was similar to the "quadruple unity" of my first break. The fabric designers it seemed to me had unconsciously moved this development forward.

In particular, right from the start and overnight, a foreign, elementary language erupted inside of me. It lay on my tongue even more naturally than our German language; and so I could speak it more quickly and can still do so. A colleague I spoke it to was reminded of Ancient Greek; a Latvian patient in the institution whom I answered in my language felt stirrings of his native country. Of course, it reminded me of the French-sounding language that had erupted from Sister H. in her dream. But I also compared it to the "speaking in tongues" which Paul talks about as a "spiritual gift." It had to have a meaning, because why would God use a meaningless language when there were understandable ones? Wasn't speaking in tongues seen as an accompanying symptom to a spiritual shock erupting from the inside, just as my language had? Didn't the driving spirit rise from the same source?

"The kingdom of heaven resides within you," Jesus said. It's just difficult to recognize something coming from within when it's so unrelated to normal experience. Words such as "epiphany" and "inspiration" wouldn't exist if such experiences weren't generally considered so foreign that one first thinks they're coming from the outside — as fed from without, as inspired, which originally meant "breathed into." Psychiatry considers thoughts and impulses that are felt to be "fed into one" as the expression of a mental split and hence speaks of "schizophrenia," which means "split soul" or "being split through mental illness."

In my erupted language I had less desire to form valid and constant sound symbols for objects and concepts than to express what was notable in the moment. This happened through a flowing language with corresponding sounds, for example, expressing with a tree the gnarly quality of its branches or the light-infused green of its leaves. And so I also became more aware of the idiosyncrasies of our German language. With a few sounds our language can express the nature of the named. The word *Baum* [tree] allows one to feel the top and its billowing body (*aum* has a round feel to it that implies the crown, with the solid B the solidity of the trunk). In English, "tree" makes me think more of a thin pine tree or a bendable sapling without the space of the crown. *Blume* [flower] sounds mysterious, resting in itself, very different from *Blüte* [blossom] in which you can hear the transition to fruit, which also has something fruity in its pithy sound. In the Biblical creation story God lets humans name what he has created. Tree, flower, blossom, fruit seemed to me words which directly let one feel the being of the created.

"In the beginning was the WORD" it says in the Gospel of John and already in the sounds or letters the MEANING is expressed. In thought I let the WORD [German Wort] be sung by children in four groups as a four-note chord and a seventh chord: in the depths the vibrating WWWWW, above it the open OOOOO, over this the rolling RRRRR, and even higher the light TTTTT. It would sound like a locomotive, like a dynamic forward-driving energy.

Sung, the WWWWW sounds like shaking waves still lacking form. A sound of movement and breadth in wind and clouds, waves and water. The spirit in the beginning. The zig-zag wave line in the W consists of two of the same components: a V and another V, negatively and positively loaded energy, a male and a female, from whose union the round world figure evolves in the O, as people believed in antiquity. As Omega, the O was the symbol for God. The R was taken from the circle, but it wasn't the entire circle but rather only held the section; in the "INRI" above the cross it stood for "Rex," for the king. In the T one then has the length and breadth of the world. TTTT sounds like the progression of units of time without a development that ties it to a before or after. Without the T the WOR only sounds like a timeless triad resting within itself. And the trinity was probably conceived with that timeless quality of resting within itself.

"I saw you passing by on the street as I looked out of the window today. You were walking so stooped," an old friend told me. Weighed down by the burden of coherences otherwise not felt — that is exactly how I felt. How exhausting it would be if one always felt it, I thought. Or one would have had to grow up with it. Nothing seemed random anymore; nothing seemed to have just one meaning without simultaneously having significance beyond this meaning. Our bodies with their many toes and fingers, the double arms and legs, the body halves, the single form of neck and head simultaneously seemed to be expressing our goal: to develop from the manifold into unity, and from unity to develop in the spiritual realm just as the tree is able to spread out its network of branches from the one trunk.

"Relation and signification ideas" is how psychiatry refers to this thinking and experiencing in symbols and comprehensive contexts of meaning: for them it's just a symptom of illness and has no further sense except that the affected, sick person is "schizophrenic." I now referred to it as "central experiencing." As with a fan, all the presentations of life which otherwise don't seem to relate to one another, reach out from a common center and are connected to it. The normal sense of the world resembles the compartment system of a desk; everything has its place but remains isolated and God too has his own compartment, the religion compartment.

A feeling of pending liberation filled me. I mean in particular the liberation from the purely negative view of psychosis, from our devaluation by psychiatry. I tore apart all my wood-bead necklaces as if they were metal chains — the chains in which we felt captured by the psychiatrists' lack of understanding. The beads jumped around the room. I collected them and put them in an empty marmalade jar. I again let my hands work on their own and observed how they filled the glass with the beads. It was like asking something of the *I Ching,* the ancient Chinese book of wisdom — the person seeking advice gives themselves over completely to the repeated movement of yarrow stems in order to find the present and future among sixty-four signs of the *Book of Changes.* On top of the last black beads my hands laid a few red ones, unfortunately only a few. When I found the closed jar many years later, I couldn't resist putting the red beads on top. But real symbolic acts as divined signs of future developments are impossible through will, but only from the instinctual impulses of the subconscious.

A Hans would help us — it came to me. Which Hans would it be? I could only think of bishop Hanns Lilje.[1] I looked into it and sent the publisher of his "Sunday Leaflet" two books about healing through faith and prayer by

1 Hanns Lilje was a German Lutheran bishop and leader of the ecumenical movement.

Agnes Sanford[2] and Rebecca Beard.[3] I included a review by a GDR female theologian I was familiar with and asked the publisher to reference the books in the "Sunday Leaflet." That Rebecca Beard, a doctor, could make the connection between body and soul understandable seemed a helpful introduction to spiritual healing. I did not receive an answer and also didn't get the books back. So, it wouldn't be Hanns Lilje.

In June of 1959 I traveled out of the country to the Barlach[4] exhibit. As I stood in the entrance hall of the Kunsthaus and walked up the broad staircase, Rodin's John the Baptist stood all alone at the top. I had previously seen him in the exhibit "Sculpture in the Open," but it was only here, surrounded by quiet, that his movement found its full expression. I was deeply moved. Like a fugue by Bach, the sculpture developed out of its counterpoint.

This was an important experience that stirred a lot inside of me. Once I was home again, I had spontaneous epiphanies upon waking for a week. It was like it was before my break in 1936. This time they were ideas related to how nature is structured.

The first morning, it was about the structure of plants, coming from a static and a dynamic element. The static element is the stem, the dynamic one is the leaf; in the blossom both return in a transformed iteration. I had never paid attention to that. Right after breakfast I compared the green leaves of flowers and bushes with the petals of their blossoms.

The next morning, I followed the structure of the human body, applying the same principle. The stem turned into bones, the leaf structure into muscle fibers. But where was the theme of the fugue that goes through

2 Agnes Sanford was an American Christian writer and proponent of the inner healing movement.

3 Rebecca Beard was an American Quaker writer and proponent of spiritual therapy.

4 Ernst Barlach was a German expressionist artist.

the entire form and connects all the partial forms with one another? I had found it in the transformed return of the green leaf in the flower petal. But I did not find it in the human body yet. Full of excitement, I waited for the next morning. In the inside of the foot I would find the theme, I knew on waking. I looked at my foot, drew the inside and then turned the drawing so that the foot stood on top of the ankle. Standing upright, the foot became a torso on its side. The big toe became the neck, the front ball of the foot became the shoulder blade, the ankle with the heel became the rump. The top and bottom of the foot's arch became the rounded abdomen and the drawn-in spine. I added a second foot to it that was turned down. Ankle and heel as rump was the same for both, the extended arch became the thigh, the front ball of the foot became the calf, and the big toe the lower leg. Now I drew a proper foot underneath it and the human made of three feet of different lengths stood before me. Hands and arms reveal a just recognizable foot that has been lengthened in the formal structure.

So there I had the epiphany of the structural laws of the human body that I had not received during my education. Without doubt the morning "epiphanies" wanted to compensate for my inadequate nude figure studies. My unconscious was helping to rebalance my shattered self-confidence.

Now it also became clear to me where the structure of the musical fugue that I had often played in Bach's little preludes came from. The fugue too varies a theme through all voices, in order to, at the end, have all the voices come in together in the *stretto* — just as with plants in the blossom and with us in head and face, all forms and colors come together in a very small space. The laws of art are unconsciously adopted from the laws of form in nature.

The fourth morning, rhythm joined the development: unity — order — central bringing together into a larger whole — central hierarchy. I first realized it with the individual plant. From the wholeness of the seed, it spreads into the root system with its rows of roots in the depths of the earth and simultaneously the stem and leaf shoots move toward the light; it is evident in the stems and leaves and finally produces the centrally organized blossoms.

In the gardens I verified this developmental rhythm, looking at leaf position and blossom placement of flowers, bushes, and trees. Whether the green leaves had fingers, as with the lupine or the horse chestnut, or whether they formed opposing pairs, as with lilacs or a rosette, or as with the plantain or the foxglove always oriented around a center, this attained center seemed to be the condition for the centrally layered petal rows which followed the green leaves.

The fifth morning, the same rhythm presented itself, in the developmental history of all of nature. In pre-historic times, the same and similar formal elements lined up next to or on top of one another, as in the case of ferns and horsetail, in the animal kingdom with the segmented animals such as tapeworms, the arthropods, and others. The fish skeleton as well, which resembles fern, reminds one, with its lined-up bones, of the early period of ordering. The vertebrae correspond with the horsetail principle. It isn't until later that the central forms of the blossom develop, and in the animal kingdom we see skulls and pelvises, and the embryo is moved inside.

In the *Health Brockhaus*[5] I looked at the developmental stages of humans. The placenta around the embryo in the amniotic sac, in which it lies protected, seems to repeat the developmental rhythm of pre-historic plants. The plantlike villi remind one in their first phase of algae

5 Helmut Mommsen, *Der Gesundheits-Brockhaus: Volksbuch vom Menschen und der praktischen Heilkunde* (Wiesbaden: Brockhaus, 1951), a physiological text.

and moss-like forms, which develop from the centrally gathered to the centrally layered.

Plant, bush, tree — here again I saw the order of what is arrayed through the centrally gathered and the centrally layered. This drive to win space seemed to be common in all beings. In mental development, the creative as well as destructive. In sacred architecture comes the initial arrangement of boulders in the North or columns in the South, which represented the multitude of gods. Later comes the central edifice of the one God with tiered towers. The same rhythm happens with missiles: from the spear, the cannonball, and the tiered skyrocket.

The sixth morning, the basic movements that generate the development rhythm revealed themselves: stretching, contracting, circling. Stretching from a whole into a series — contracting to a larger whole of a central form — stretching in space as layers which through circling movements become spirals. Later I found the first forms of life depicted in a plant book: stick-formed, ball-formed, and spiral bacteria. They seemed to me to be arch-representatives of the basic movements which they expressed in their form: stretching in the stick form, contracting in the ball form, and circling in the spirals.

I was familiar with form as a result of the movements of making pottery on the wheel, and from sculpting. But with those it was my movement that determined the form. That every figure was the result of a dominating inner movement was something I was only now beginning to sense. We execute the same movements with our bodies. It's not only our joints and muscles that reflect the three basic movements — stretching, contracting, and circling.

I got the impression that everything sentient, all physical and mental development, is directed by the constant change of direction in movement — starting with the back-and-forth between sleeping (contracting) and wakefulness (stretching). This movement goes all the way into how styles of art develop over time periods, in that more inwardly focused forms of expression switch off with forms that are oriented more toward the outside.

The seventh morning, the structure of the universe followed the same rhythm of progressing development and order: unity — expansion of the gases — attraction and contracting to larger units of the galaxies — expansion of these systems in the universe, comparable with the tiered flower heads. The star systems of the galaxies that rotate around a center, created by smaller units; the planetary systems that circle around their sun, rotating in even smaller units; the orb of individual planets, seemed to me like the symbol of our developmental aim: a great, central circling WE, in which the I of the individual orb remains completely intact.

After getting up I opened the little encyclopedia and found the illustration of a globular cluster that contradicts this development and progression rhythm. The basic unit is the globe, the larger unit is again globular and the distribution of the globular cluster around our Milky Way forms a ball. That reminded me of the repetition of the same and similar forms among plants and animals in prehistoric times. The globular clusters apparently didn't rotate anymore, or did so weakly, otherwise they couldn't be ball shaped. But didn't they at some point rotate? Would they have otherwise formed these kinds of units? Everything begins moving. Life began in moving water. We too started in amniotic fluid and were born into the world as kicking babies. Were the globular clusters the old ones of the universe that had lost their rotating movement around their center?

I was drawn to visit the water on this morning. And there, as if hit by a lightning bolt, I was overcome with the terrible certainty: a great chill was coming. Snow and ice covered the earth. The "last judgment" had turned into the "last green judgment": from now on there would be no judgment, no more green judgment, because there was no more warmth to allow the leaves and fruit to grow. Suddenly a thought grabbed me: humans are doing this to themselves. The great chill arrived because we hadn't stuck to the development principle.

I was devastated. The sun would dim—I couldn't explain the great chill any other way. I thought of Jesus's word about the end of the world and his reappearance when "sun and moon lose their glow and stars fall from heaven,"[6] before Christ returns "into the clouds of heaven with great power and glory."[7] Previously I could only explain this prediction from my worldview that put earth at the center, circled by the sun; nothing indicates that Jesus didn't share this worldview. According to the Biblical genesis story, God created the world and its creatures like a sculptor, hadn't let them evolve in interminably long periods of time as we assume today. One had to think he could finish them off just as suddenly.

Now I was overcome by the thought that Jesus had always been among us and shared our lives in many forms. He was not the prophesied world judge, he was our brother. He was among us in Johann Sebastian Bach and in Vincent van Gogh, who doubted himself. And now he was in me, the "mentally ill" woman, the forcibly sterilized woman. And so he was also affected by my sterilization: he couldn't be reborn.

Deeply disturbed, I sent my sister in Bonn a letter by express mail that she must inform the government about the approaching great chill. I also wrote that there would be a solar eclipse, that Jesus had always been among us and was now affected by my forcible sterilization as well.

I wrote to my professor that he should stock up on enough coals and food supplies. Dried peas warmed better than rice, I added. I had the notion that the great chill

6 Cf. Matthew 24:29.
7 Cf. Matthew 24:30.

would last a long time. The summer of 1959 turned out to be very hot — my letter must have seemed very strange.

I'd lacked a sense of time in March of 1936 when I was overcome with the certainty of an approaching "terrible" war. I'd also thought it was imminent; in reality it didn't break out for another three-and-a-half years. This time it wasn't about a war. By now we know that the end of life on earth will not happen through God or the forces of nature but through humans, when the weapons that can annihilate all of life are not destroyed. We know that a chain of atomic explosions can make the sun disappear behind a dense cloud of dust, smoke, and ash, and cause a long, enduring chill. And we know that the stored atom bombs can also be detonated by a chain of coincidences. I still don't believe that my certainty, which overcame me as powerfully as lightning, was ridiculous. Only my reactions were ridiculous — back then my insufficient attempts to stop the war, and this time my fantasies about the reason for the approaching great chill.

In spite of my idea that Jesus had always lived among us and was now in me, I was nonetheless filled by the Biblical promise of his return "in the clouds of heaven with great power and glory." I saw the shining golden Viking ship with full white sails appearing against the green evening sky and approaching fast followed by a swarm of little boats with colored sails. Gently they landed on the earth in front of the doors of those who wanted to join them. And there were many who wanted to join and sail with them: it wasn't just the "chosen" who, according to Matthew and Mark, are gathered by the angels of the Lord "by the four winds from the end of earth to the end of heaven." The little boats swayed toward the great ship under the weight of their burden. There was room for everyone.

"There comes a ship loaded / up to the highest hold / carries God's son full of grace, / the father's eternal word" — the promise of this old church song was literally becoming reality. And then the captain stepped up to the bow of the ship, stretched out his arm, and boomed: "Sun, follow our trail!" And the sun accompanied the ship through the cold of the universe to a new world. So that is why the sun lost its shine for a while. That is why it would become cold during this time. To believe that now was not difficult at all for me. Whoever created the world can also change it, I told myself. Collecting physically real humans through spiritual angels "of the four winds" seemed more difficult to me. The colored sails replaced the angel wings.

When a few days later, after midnight, there was a ring at the bell and two policemen and a doctor from the health service stood in front of the door, I threw the key-chain at the doctor's chest. There he was in the middle of the night with policemen as if to get a criminal! He disappeared right away without talking to me. In the hallway, I showed the two policemen the page in the Book of Matthew about the return of Christ in my brass-bound Bible. "It will happen soon!" I said with full conviction. When they laughed, I threw the Bible to the floor with such rage that the brass fitting bent. I picked it up again and led the policemen into the living room of my landlady, who thankfully was traveling. I offered them tea because it would take a while for me to get dressed.

The express letter had worried my sister. Since she couldn't come herself, she'd called the health service—without having any idea that the service would call in the police to help. In the end I had to be thankful that they came at night; this way hardly any of the other renters would see me being picked up by the police.

During the admission interview in the institution, I told the nice young female doctor I had to give credence to the lightning-like certainty that came over me of an approaching chill. During my first break in spring of 1936, I'd been overcome with the same force by the certainty of an approaching "terrible" war, which broke out three-

and-a-half-years later. I was still deeply disturbed. The doctor listened to me empathetically. But right after our conversation — I was now lying in bed in the sleeping hall — she came with a sedative injection. That was the only answer that institution doctors knew to provide us in response to our experiences.

I lay in the large admission hall with a number of rows of beds. The female patients lay next to each other one bed after the other, only separated by a nightstand. All of them were sedated with injections. I hadn't experienced that yet: that we should be incapacitated with psychotropic drugs right after being admitted and then kept sedated. In a brief time, we were also so physically weakened that I stumbled to the bathroom on unstable legs. I had to hold onto the edge of the bed in order not to fall. My hand trembled so much that I could hardly hold the cup and spilled my coffee.

"Stop making a scene!" the young nurse barked at a female patient who buckled on her way to the bathroom. That was the most eerie part of what I experienced in the institution: a large hall full of intentionally weakened, half- or fully sedated patients. The doctors barely knew what was going on, what they were experiencing, but they had the authority to take our last bit of freedom in a locked house: the freedom of our thoughts, our consciousness, and our bodies.

Even if we were put into duration baths in Bethel in 1936, or got sedative injections, once we woke, we were fully present again and not weakened physically. We didn't have to swallow our fear and our resistance but could express them anew. Is this forced silence really progress from the "restless wards," with their justified resistance against psychiatric methods, which fight and devalue the patient and their experiences?

I protested against the forced injections, I tried to explain that my previous break had receded on its own without medication and had actually led to a break-free period of thirteen years. The medication-induced interruption of the psychosis had led to new outbreaks after just five and three years. None of it helped. "Just leave it to us," one of the doctors in the admission ward said. "We can already see what is going on with you." The experience of the patient and the meaning it has for them didn't interest our psychiatrists. They were only interested in the symptoms and behavior that deviated from the NORM. The power of these psychiatrists to force their limited viewpoint on us with medication is frightening for us.

Luckily, I got a rash after three days so that the injections had to be stopped. Instead, the nurse now stuffed pills in my mouth. I had to suffer it, but she didn't force me to swallow them, as is done nowadays. I kept them under my tongue and waited for an opportunity to flush them down the toilet when nobody was looking. None of the doctors noticed that from that time, until about eight weeks later when I was discharged, I had not been medicated. Prior to being discharged I told the ward doctor that I had never swallowed pills. "We have to treat with medication," he noted, "insurance demands it of us."

We weren't taken seriously. In vain I tried to explain to the female chief physician during rounds in the admission ward that while I experienced my impulses as an inner voice, I didn't hear voices. She insisted: I was hearing voices.

In the next row of beds diagonally from me there lay a woman of about thirty. From what she said I figured out she was a hotel cook. Overwhelmed by her psychosis experience, she quietly mumbled continuously. She had only just been admitted and not sedated. Her self-talk indicated that even things that seemed irrelevant to me now were creating meaningful coherence for her. She had clearly experienced a conversion. Repeatedly, the astonished sentence broke out from her randomly: "It's all perfectly clear."

Her monologues were so quiet that she actually couldn't bother anyone. But the nurses had to silence her no matter what. She defended herself. The nurses fastened her to the bed with leather belts and forced sedative injections on her. *What* she said was of no interest; nobody had listened to her. That she spoke, even if it was quiet, was against the institution norms and was sufficient to tie her to the bed and to suffocate with medication the for-her substantive experience of meaningful contexts in her life. Even after her discharge she'll hardly have a chance to talk to someone about her psychosis events. It never seemed to be worth the doctors' and nurses' time to try to understand or even to listen to what we patients had gone through.

The education of young nurses was more inadequate in this institution than any of the others I had been in. The nurses' and health aides' behavior reveals how institution directors and doctors feel about their patients. I had not encountered such openly contemptuous treatment as I did here. The doctors knew about it because we complained, but they didn't change anything. It seems very important to me that doctors and care personnel know how unforgettably good or bad institutional treatment imprints in us. But as care personnel must induce patients into partial or full sedation, it's hard to recognize the patient as a fully equal, fellow human being. This type of work can't make one happy. How enriching would it be, by contrast, for those interested in psychology to listen carefully and talk to psychotic patients.[8]

The half-open ward into which I was moved wasn't much better. Here too, there was a stifling lack of space in large sleeping halls, which simultaneously served as a day room and dining hall. Here I realized the four institu-

8 Buck commented to her friend and publisher Fritz Bremer, as he related it to me, that she felt the psychiatric system "brutalized" those working in it as well as those caught in it.

tions I'd previously experienced had all had an especially good reputation and seemed to be the exceptions. This mass institution, with its uncaring lodging of patients without any kind of occupation, was more the rule in our FRG institutions in 1959 and far into the 1960s and '70s.

"In the past, this institution would have included a large farm and workshops, a weaving plant, cobbler's workshop, basket weaving workshop and others," an older nurse explained to me. Apparently, the only thing remaining was the basket-weaving workshop. Even the long-term patients were now just put under medication.

For the first time, however, we tried to help ourselves on this ward. The summer of 1959 was very hot, so we were allowed to stay in the little ward garden most of the time. A group of about eight female patients sat on recliners that were shoved together and talked about what had struck us most during our psychosis experiences. This way we could give one another confirmation of the meaning of our experience and separate ourselves from the devaluing psychiatric evaluation that undermined our confidence. These hot summer days, above us the crowns of the pines in whose shadows we discussed our psychosis and dreams in a relaxed way, and thought about them, belong to my good memories of my time in institutions. It is the fellow patients through whom institutional time becomes rewarding, because they have known what psychosis is and know more about it than specialists. The specialists neither have the experiences themselves, nor are willing to learn about them by talking to their patients.

For a female patient in her first break who only heard individual sentences, it was still impossible to see a meaning in them; she couldn't understand the context and connection. Those of us who had experienced a number of breaks and thus had more comprehensive psychosis experiences found it easier to recognize the meaning.

A female patient who'd already had a number of breaks wrote down what happened in her psychosis and gave the notes to the female ward doctor. She'd hoped for the explanation that would help her understand it. But as a response she only got: "Well, that's all very nice." The doctor was friendly and empathetic; if she had been able to say something about understanding this she would surely have tried. But our universities simply don't provide the appropriate education.

This patient told me about experiences of everything unifying. She much later read about similar events in the biography of an East Indian. She was a woman with a simple background, and she could hardly have known about the book. Aside from such happy experiences, she had a compulsion to add up people's value by the numerical value of the letters of their names. Where nothing could exist without meaning, even names had to have a secret meaning. In the book *Mysticism and Magic of Numbers* by F.C. Endres I later read,[9] as I found out about psychoanalysis, that this same transformation of letters into number values and vice-versa had occurred two hundred years earlier among Kabbalistic scholars. That it is much older may be indicated by Roman letters that represent number values. If this patient could have seen such parallels, then she could have understood her compulsive behavior better: a breaking open of "archaic idea possibilities," as happens in schizophrenia according to C.G. Jung. Perhaps they would then have lost their compulsiveness for her. What one understands affords one more freedom.

I told this fellow patient how I had transformed WORD into a sung tetrachord. And this she found quite strange, for children to transform WORD into a steam piston and jet-propelled sound, and now also a symbol of a unity of four. Schizophrenics amongst one another....

9 Franz Carl Endres, *Mystiek und Magie der Zahlen* (Zurich: Rascher, 1951).

In the little garden of this half-open ward, we also had fun with movement games we'd played as children: "Green light go," "Mother, how many steps can I take?" The young nurse who watched us outside was invited to join us. She refused. Apparently, she'd been instructed to keep her distance and to only talk about the most necessary things with us.

We female patients had a good community characterized by empathy and a willingness to help. I have known this self-understood solidarity during most of the times I was in institutions. The psychiatric teaching of "schizophrenics without contact" is the result of a prejudice. It does not do justice to the way we are with one another.

As I lay in the ward garden, I felt an expression of tender care in every branch and every leaf in the bushes. They seemed to express the spirit of the creator, the quiet unfolding, the slow development of everything living on earth just as directly as a work of art reflects the spirit of the artist.

It became clear to me that the outbreak of ideas in my psychosis was in reaction to what previously happened. The morning insights into the structure of nature were an answer to my insecurity, after I recognized I wasn't sufficiently prepared for my profession due to the missing study of nudes. The human-induced "last green day of judgment" was an answer to my doubt about the promised "judgment day," with the reward of heaven and the punishment of hell. It was part of my longtime questioning of the idea that a loving Father-God could really judge and punish rather than letting us recognize our mistakes ourselves. The idea that Jesus had always been among us related to conversations with my friend at school, who said: "He should have modeled a life for us, as husband, as father, he should have grown old."

I connected this to the fate of my life. The mythical picture that Jesus was in me and suffered from my forcible sterilization because he couldn't be reborn also expressed my pain on account of this act, which I'd been surprised with in, of all things, the "City of God" Bethel. I revised what he had said in the promise of judgment: "What you have or have not done to the least of my brothers (and sisters), you have or have not done to me."[10] The idea of his return "with great power and glory" I clearly couldn't give up without having experienced it in my imagination. That the little boats had not just taken the "chosen" with them was another answer to my doubts regarding a godly court of judgment.

Wasn't the fact that the outbreak of ideas answered something previous also proof that they came from inside, even though I'd experienced them as having been "given from the outside?" Didn't the morning insights about the structure of nature from a few basic movements and a diversely varied form-theme allow one to conclude that we carry the laws of nature unconsciously in ourselves, and this unconscious knowledge can move into the conscious through the outbreak of impulses? Did these impulses also prepare one to have other psychosis content become conscious? These questions now occupied me.

During the medical exit interview in the open house in which I'd last been held, the ward doctor said something about the morning insights into the structure of nature. "That isn't sick," he countered. That is how our experiences can be pushed aside in a two-fold way: either because they are "sick" or because they are "not sick." The psychiatrist was only interested in symptoms; whatever is not clearly recognizable as "sick" in his eyes has nothing to do with the psychosis. In this way he can continue to maintain his opinion that psychosis is a meaningless occurrence: the connection between symptom and history is randomly ripped apart.

10 Cf. Matthew 25:40.

For me, this connection was directly understandable. For me, my psychotic break didn't begin with the certainty of an approaching chill and my reactions to it, but rather weeks earlier with the breaking open of impulses that started off as weak ones. In the invasion of the approaching chill, the impulses had simply gotten much stronger. I saw the psychosis as a process of development and stuck to my opinion even against the doctors. But this made little sense to them. They could not recognize it, because they didn't have conversations with us and didn't take us seriously.

This open house with smaller rooms and its own dining room was good. The nurses were nice here, too. We only saw the professor rushing by when he went to the private ward.

Our psychoses had receded. My fellow patients had been suppressed with psychotropic drugs, in my case, the break had receded without medication. We had grown our thick skin back, the close community began to disintegrate. I felt again the slow abatement of the strong impulses of the acute break into just a quiet instinct, as with the previous break, which had also not been interrupted with medication.

We were close to being discharged.

10

Deep in Growth

After being discharged, I noticed my night dreams had stopped since the opening of the psychotic break. Or had I just forgotten them by morning? I could only explain it to myself by the thought that the psychotic ideas had taken the place of night dreams; and so they must have been coming from the same source; from my own unconscious. The French-sounding language of Sister H., which had broken out from her nightly dreams as she went into psychosis, already put me on that trail. Psychotic ideas are as visual as dreams, in contrast to the abstract thinking of the normal consciousness. Just as little as a dream is the sign of a mental illness, the psychotic idea is, I told myself. Our illness can only lie in the fact that we confuse our psychosis with reality, which we do in dreams only as long as we are dreaming. If I understood the ideas of my receded psychosis on the dream level, they lost their absolute character of reality but could still keep their meaning. And they didn't seem real to me anymore once I returned to a normal state. With my earlier breaks, I couldn't understand afterward that I could have believed such fantastical things. This time it was different: I now understood that in the psychosis experience one was dealing with a symbolic reality.

This understanding of psychosis on the dream level had something deeply satisfying for me. Now I was finally completely immune against the devaluation by the psychiatric prejudice that schizophrenia was a physically caused, genetically contingent, and incurable mental illness. When I speak to other individuals today about our schizophrenic experience it's evident how impressive these experiences of an altered state of being were and are for everyone, and how little the negative judgment of psychiatry can do them justice. But as long as we don't recognize the symbolic character of these experiences and look at them in the same way as we see normal everyday reality, we can hardly escape the psychiatric devaluation.

It's probably on account of this negative judgment that many affected individuals experience their psychosis as something frightening. Many also fall into panic because they are afraid of being "mentally ill," having to be admitted to an institution, losing a partner, friends, and a job. When, between my fourth and fifth break, I was once again depressed about being marked as "mentally ill" and about my forced sterilization, my oldest sister said almost impatiently: "But that's only a relative evaluation. In antiquity the mentally ill were honored as being especially close to the gods." Never had anyone before told me anything so encouraging. Even today, decades later, I remember exactly what part of the path we were on where she said that.

It became clear to me that a cure was only possible through an understanding of the broken-open unconscious and its inclusion in the conscious. I started to separate the meaningful from the ridiculous, but tried to keep the receding, now much-weaker impulses by paying attention to and following them in everything I did. I felt more alive through them and more secure even with the most quotidian things. I wished to remain thus unified with the whole. I told myself: if you never suppress your unconscious again but live out of your impulses, it won't have to open up in a new break as a dammed energy. That is why it was so important for me not to suppress my final break with medication, because this way I could, as with my previous break, keep the impulses.

The last impulse to inexplicable action, even to me, that I remember was in April 1961. Early in the morning I had the urge — in a jogging suit over my nightgown — to replant a larkspur from one flower bed to another in my garden. Why, I didn't know myself. There was something in the air that demanded this expression. Back in bed and listening to the morning news I found out that on this morning Gagarin[1] left for space. A typical schizophrenic symbolic act, to accompany the beginning of space exploration with the replanting of a larkspur from one flower bed to another. It had to be a larkspur![2]

Then, in spite of all attempts to retain the instinct, that morning I waited in vain for it. Now I had to again find my way in a normal state. But I'd liberated myself from the psychiatric devaluing. I was sure that a purely negative evaluation had to be wrong.

A morning sequence of "broken open memories from early childhood," as I named them this week, put a final end to my psychosis. I think it was in November of 1959. This symbolic childhood replaced everything for me that I had done without in reality. I experienced it on a different planet, where everything was further developed than on earth. The last morning of this sequence my father returned home — he had dark skin like an African — from one of his weeklong space travels. When I was younger, he'd sometimes taken me on these space trips. He used a lens-shaped, transparent model of the galaxy with different-colored points to explain that the points were animated planets and the different colors indicated each

1 Yuri Gagarin, Russian cosmonaut, launched into space on April 12, 1961.

2 The German word for larkspur, *Rittersporn*, literally means "knight's spur."

one's respective stage of development. He was a specialist on everything that rotated. At home he was a carousel and music-box builder.

This morning I was eighteen but behaved like a child. I sat in the middle of my dolls and teddy bears and didn't let his return bother me. "If only you would grow up!" he said, disgruntled. I continued to play unperturbed. Then he was lying on the floor to get balls out from under the cupboards under which he'd let them roll. "I have an idea I'd like to talk to you about," he said. He often discussed his thoughts with me, but never such a thought. "I think we should separate for a while. I want to send you where you will become a grownup." — "And the lamb?" was all I asked. He'd given me a little lamb that I loved very much. "You get to take the lamb with you." I hoped he wouldn't succeed at catching the lively lamb, but he did succeed, and we both disappeared.

On this morning I got up with wobbly knees. I was deeply shocked that I could have treated my loving father in such a manner. Could that have been reality? My banishment from paradise to earth which was this place of growing up?

The next and last morning of this sequence of experiences the father who'd accompanied me through the fantasized childhood revealed himself to be a psychotherapist. After the shock of the previous morning, I was very relieved about this. He walked away smiling at me until we couldn't see each other anymore. Now I knew that everything had been a game or psychotherapy, but that didn't take away from the healing effect of this love-filled childhood. Now I had also fully accepted myself as a child and had experienced myself as being loved. Just one week, for one or two hours in the morning after waking up. But that was enough. The intensity of the experience is clearly more important than its duration. Now I felt cured.[3]

In the following weeks, I expanded on this childhood with games and encounters and activities which the completely different circumstances on that faraway planet brought out. Finally, it turned into a full-blown childhood story. For a long time it had the same value as my real childhood, whose experiences spread over many years and so were not as present as the events, or at least the spirit, of my made-up childhood.

I wasn't quite convinced that the cohesive morning sequence could have been only a product of my own unconscious. Didn't there have to be someone behind this who knew that this experience was necessary for me? But if it did arise from my unconscious, that was proof of the equalizing and healing nature of that unconscious. Psychosis was an attempt at healing, just as many symptoms of physical illnesses are attempts at healing. And as a healing—not just as liberation from being devalued as a mentally ill woman—I had also experienced it in my breaks.

The morning insights in the meaning of the basic movements woke my interest in nature. In a popular science book, I read with amazement that if all the atoms in our bodies were closely packed together they wouldn't even cover a pinhead. Everything else was just space, space for the movement of electrons switching from their inner to outer orbits and vice-versa, circling around an atomic nucleus made of protons and neutrons. Our physics and chemistry teachers had studied before Niels Bohr developed his atomic model and won the Nobel Prize in 1922; they'd told us nothing of the atomic structure of matter. With this dynamic structure of matter, it seemed only logical to me that basic movements had as important a

3 Buck would tell filmmaker Alexandra Pohlmeier later in life of her psychosis, "I miss it."

role as basic substances did. Wasn't the essential already present in the atom? Quiet in the nucleus and movement in the circling electrons, heavy and light, positive and negative load—everywhere a harmonic interplay of opposing forces. Like an atomic family from which the many differing forms of the world have developed.

In May 1960,[4] I moved into a studio with a little garden. Now I could observe the growth of sown summer flowers from the moment their first seed leaf appeared. This first and second seed leaf seemed important to me relative to the later form of the flower, and for the contrast of the stronger and weaker forms. In cosmos, which develop needle-fine leaves and then a broad-leafed flower, the form seemed to fall back on its first seed leaf's shape. By contrast, the hollyhock's first seed leaf is already serrated, as are its later leaves; the lack of a primitive seed leaf leads to the conclusion there won't be great contrasts in form in the developed plant. The sunflower, with its strongly contrasting form, seems to fall back on the long shape of its second seed leaf as it flowers, while the broad green leaves correspond with the primitive first seed leaf.

After recovering I tried to gain more clarity about the nature of psychosis. I wrote a number of essays about it. Since none of the numerous psychiatrists I'd known could tell us anything to understand psychosis, I had the impression that I was closer to the truth than they were. I looked at the unconscious for the basis of psychosis and our understanding it at the dream level. Now I tried to determine whether others had had these insights before me. I found Theodor Bovet's book *The Human Being: Their Illnesses and Changes.*[5] While it was about neuroses, not psychoses, Bovet's opinion that psychiatry had "landed

4 Buck would live in her "garden cottage" in Hamburg for the next forty years.

5 Theodor Bovet, *Die Person: Ihre Krankheiten und Wandlungen* (Tübingen: Katzmann-Verlag, 1948). Bovet was a Swiss neurologist and counselor.

in a one-way street" encouraged me. At the end of May 1960, I sent him an essay called "Development and Course of Psychosis" and asked him whether my views made sense to him.

Bovet answered: "Your views are absolutely correct but they have already been adopted by a few psychiatrists for about the last ten years. The idea that mental illnesses, especially schizophrenia, should be treated spiritually through empathy and analysis of the unconscious was, by the way, developed by a non-medical person, Mrs. Sechehaye[6] in Geneva, who realized this with a female patient. Since then there have been a series of cases that are known (Prof. Benedetti, Basel; Dr. Chr. Müller, Zurich; and Dr. Siirala, Zurich among others). Except this treatment currently requires about one doctor per patient so that it is not broadly applicable."

Bovet's letter encouraged me. Now I had to think about the question of whether the understanding of psychosis couldn't be treated "broadly." Group conversations seemed like a good option to me; our conversations in the institution garden had been a beginning. It had helped my own understanding very much to formulate my psychosis experiences and to summarize them in essays: I won distance by having them in front of me in written form. In a group, a similar effect should be attainable if patients worked together on a "primer of schizophrenia." When someone confronts and works on what bothers them, they can develop from it. I imagined this primer as a picture book with short captions. Every group would develop a new one, it would be different every time, until a summary of all the essentials could be published, taken from the primers or short notes from individual affected individuals. It would be a basic primer of schizophrenia that could give orientation and a deeper self-understand-

6 Marguerite Sechehaye was a Swiss psychoanalyst who treated schizophrenia with psychoanalysis.

ing to psychiatry patients who were in clinics or institutions.

Because, in spite of the great differences in psychosis content, the basic pattern still seems to be similar. With everyone, clearly a spiritual conflict, a life crisis, or a heavy burden preceded a break, which they tried to overcome in vain until a limit was reached beyond which they couldn't continue. With the psychosis, an energy breaks out that takes charge. Certainly, every schizophrenic has the feeling of not thinking or acting as themselves anymore. Thinking of a person's own volition is replaced by "provided," sometimes also "withdrawn" thoughts; acting as oneself is replaced by inner impulses or "voices," which don't just accompany the affected and their actions in an evaluating and commenting way, but also tell them what they are supposed to do. The sense of the world is thus fundamentally changed: the broken-open psychosis content seems forcefully to be a believable reality.

The penetration of this other reality behind the known one elicits deep fears in many of the affected. The loss of self-control can feel frightening when one's own will fights it. I didn't have these fears because what happened in psychosis was more convincing to me than the normal state, which was determined by my own will. For a psychotic to understand, it's important they recognize the psychotic experiences as coming from inside. Otherwise, the schizophrenic patient feels either persecuted, or as if they were the chosen object of their "epiphanies" and "influences," without a possibility of doubting and working through this time self-critically. If, for example, the voices say something negative about the patient, it's more frightening than it is when they know the voices are coming out of themselves, and they must think about what could have affected their own self-confidence so much.

It is, however, not enough to just tell the patient: "Your psychosis experience is coming from inside of you." If it were easy to recognize that, we could tell it to ourselves. Dreams can be a bridge to understanding; and some affected in fact feel their psychosis as a kind of dream. Our unconscious uses the same resources in psychosis as it does in dreams. In the dream, too, symbols play a large role. In dreams, too, we can identify with symbols that move us or with individuals; the persons who appear in dreams usually refer to ourselves. But it's only recognizable that schizophrenia is an attempt at solving a life crisis when it's seen in the context of the person's previous history. The patient would have to have so much trust in our psychiatric system's readiness to understand them that they'd be willing to talk about the conflicts and crises that preceded their psychosis. If their psychosis is simply suppressed with medication they cannot have this trust, since they must think their experiences are being evaluated as sick and ridiculous.

It's surely easier to find in group conversations the insight into the nature of our unconscious soul that's necessary for the schizophrenic patient, in its tendencies and ways of expression. It's easier to find this in the diverse psychosis experiences of participants than in one-on-one conversations. In addition to processing their own psychosis, patients can provide important guidance for psychosis research. It would be encouraging to feel specialists are treating them with respect and recognizing their experience; their self-confidence could also grow in group conversations.

In his book, Bovet recommended reading C.G. Jung. That's how I found Jung. Already in 1912, Jung recognized schizophrenia as the breaking in of the unconscious into the conscious and in his book *Psychology of the Unconscious*[7]

7 Carl G. Jung, *Wandlungen und Symbole der Libido: Beiträge zur Entwicklungsgeschichte des Denkens* (Leipzig and Vienna: Franz Deuticke, 1912). The fourth revised edition was renamed *Symbole der Wandlung: Analyse des Vorspiels zu einer Schizophrenie*, ed. Jolande Jacobi (Zurich: Rascher Verlag, 1952). An English translation was pub-

presented the meaning of irrupting symbols. I was very distraught that our psychiatrists had refused for decades to acknowledge these insights of Freud and Jung's psychoanalysis and continued to insist on their theory of the meaningless, genetically caused somatic state. We paid for their hanging on to an errant opinion in the form of sterilization. Today, still, contemporary psychiatry textbooks contain hardly anything about fundamental psychoanalytic insights.

C.G. Jung writes in *Psychology of the Unconscious:*

> A consistent regression means a reconnection with the world of natural instinct, which in formal, i.e. idealistic views, represents the primal stuff/matter. If this can be caught by the consciousness, it will experience a rejuvenation and new restructuring. Should the consciousness prove it can't assimilate the contents of the unconscious breaking in, a dangerous situation arises in which the new contents retain their original, chaotic, and archaic form and thus explode the unity of the consciousness. The resulting mental disruption then is significantly called schizophrenia, which means being 'split' into insanity.[8]

With the retention of the "archaic form" Jung means taking symbols literally. My identification with the Biblical symbol of "the bride of Christ" was an example of that. Only through identification with the symbol had I recognized I had to develop my own nature; if I'd been able to recognize the meaning of the symbol for myself rather than identifying with the "bride of Christ," I could have

lished as *Psychology of the Unconscious: A Study of the Transformations and Symbolisms of the Libido: A Contribution to the History of the Evolution of Thought,* trans. Beatrice M. Hinkle (New York: Moffat, Yard and Company, 1916), without, however, including the afterword that Buck cites from.

8 Jung, *Symbole der Wandlung,* 703–4.

integrated it without mental disruption. The common interpretation of the "bride of Christ" as an expression of the "community of the saintly," by contrast, meant nothing to me. I believe we aren't supposed to be saintly but natural. The striving for sainthood has a catch that couldn't be overlooked in Bethel. To want to live according to a certain ideal of what we should be leads easily to inner dishonesty, because we can only really be what we are from the inside, what we have received from God as our nature. Schizophrenia, in fact, offers us a chance to experience our own nature through the "reconnection with the world of natural instincts." One should help the affected "to assimilate the contents of the unconscious as they break in," so that a "rejuvenation and new restructuring" becomes possible.

An example of growth through schizophrenia with empathetic psychotherapeutic help comes from the moving report of Gaetano Benedetti about the 1954 treatment of his patient Otto Lehner. The story is in Martti Siirala's 1961 book *Schizophrenia of the Individual and the Collective.* At the end of his therapy, Otto Lehner says:

> I find myself deep in growth now.... Today while sleeping I again wandered through my whole life. I summarized my development bit by bit. It was as if I were going through a labyrinth and was now finding everything in the right context. Yesterday some things were still loose, there a bolt, over there a nail; today everything is in its place, the clock face is whole and attached.[9]

C.G. Jung writes in *Psychology of the Unconscious:*

9 Martti Siirala, *Die Schizophrenie des Einzelnen und der Allgemeinheit* (Göttingen: Vandenhoeck & Ruprecht, 1961), 51.

> Our culture has forgotten long ago thinking symbolically, and even the theologian doesn't know how to apply the hermeneutics of the church fathers anymore... But for our patients in this situation, it can be lifesaving when the doctor uses such techniques and makes the alluded-to meaning available to the patient. In this way he makes it possible for the latter to at least assimilate a piece of the unconscious and thus by same measure break down the dangerously threatening dissociation. Simultaneously, assimilation protects the unconscious from the dangerous isolation of anyone who is confronted with an incomprehensible, irrational part of their personality. For the loneliness leads to panic and that only too often starts the next psychosis...Whoever...wants to treat this kind of dissociation must unavoidably know something about the anatomy and developmental history of the mental faculties they are about to try to cure. One demands the doctor who treats physical illnesses to know about anatomy, physiology, embryology and the comparable developmental history.[10]

The difference in the evaluation and treatment of schizophrenic patients in our institutional psychiatry is obvious. For Jung and Benedetti, the patient's *experiences* are the contents of their psychosis and the history and meaning derived from them are essential. Healing consists of making the meaning of their experience available to the patient so they can integrate it into their consciousness. Our German psychiatrists content themselves with observing symptoms and registering a behavior that deviates from the norm ("We can already see what's wrong with you"). Psychosis is generally only suppressed with medication—and also with force. That's why one

10 Jung, *Symbole der Wandlung*, 765–67.

must talk about creating "inconspicuousness" and not "healing."

In 1974, a psychiatric evaluator explained to me, after I noted I'd already been healed for fifteen years by understanding my psychosis: "There is no cure, just a suppression of symptoms." The suppression of psychosis experience through medication, possibly with force and without help processing it, can only effect "a suppression of symptoms." It's due to the psychiatrists when there's no cure, because they leave their patients without the help that is necessary and possible.

Which schizophrenic patient of ours can claim, as Otto Lehner did, "I find myself deep in growth now?" Growth through the understanding of meaning isn't promoted by suppression with medication, rather, it is nipped in the bud. "Pills rather than conversations! Pills rather than therapy!" have been for a long time the unheard complaints of psychiatric patients.

A report an affected woman recently sent me says: "My second outpatient visit with the neurologist... quietly shoved a typed manuscript about my psychotic experiences away with a pencil; the clinic where I later mentioned the manuscript due to lack of time and said they could request it from the previous treater, never requested it." This shoving away with a pencil — to even touch the report was apparently an imposition — is certainly typical of the way patient experiences are ignored. But how do psychiatrists want to understand what schizophrenia is when they don't open up to the psychosis experience? And how are patients supposed to trust them when they notice specialists who can supposedly help them don't even try to understand?

Almost eighty years ago the insight came that the psychotic content, as a breaking in of the unconscious into the conscious, has a meaning that can and must be understood. In which other area would it be possible that such fundamental knowledge would be ignored for decades?

Also, that reforms in practices such as work therapy with all patients, introduced by Hermann Simon in 1923, aren't compulsory? There is no office in our FRG that represents the issues and interests of patients; their needs continue to remain ignored. Nobody is responsible or can be held accountable for the fact that innumerable long-term patients are "shut down" with medication and forced to waste away without work or occupation. And this even happens with the danger of their becoming demented, because in the Bethel *Textbook of Mental and Neurological Medical Care* from 1975 it says: "After examinations by Grahmann, Boeters and Moeltgen and also following our own observations it is probable that long-term high doses of neuroleptics can also lead to dementia."[11]

This stubborn ignoring of insights that were made long ago put the stamp of incurable mental illness on us and surrendered us to discrimination. Whoever is marked with this stain can't reveal they're affected, and thus they have no chance to openly criticize the situation in institutions, and the institutions' refusal to effectively help. Only in meeting centers can former patients express their resentment and resignation in words such as: "Every craftsman must understand their profession, the psychiatrist doesn't need to." But not just those affected are condemned by the stigma of silence. The survivors of the "euthanasia" institutions and the four hundred thousand forcibly sterilized also couldn't and can't, even decades after the end of national socialist rule, out themselves as being affected—aside from the few who were able to convince people they were incorrectly diagnosed. To the present day, the medical profession has done no public rehabilitation; the sterilization law of 1933 was not annulled.

11 Kasper Jaspersen, *Lehrbuch der Geistes- und Nervenkrankenpflege*, 7th ed. (Bethel bei Bielefeld: Verlagshandlung der Anstalt Bethel, 1975).

Significant to the situation of patients in the psychiatric system today is the letter four Catholic and Protestant clinic pastors wrote to the clinic director of the psychiatric university clinic in Munich, Prof. Dr. Hanns Hippius on December 10, 1989: "In our encounters with patients of this clinic we frequently experience behavior of assimilation and submissiveness, even subservience toward all psychiatric institutions and persons. We feel their worries and fears regarding disciplinary measures in the case of disobedience and refusal."

It is the combination of psychiatric power and lack of insight into the nature and meaning of psychosis that makes the patient who is locked up, often forcibly, and pumped full of medication, so fearful. Who among us doesn't know this fear? In 1936 in Bethel, we were still able to protest against this inhumane safekeeping. Today's patients can't do that because they are put under medication on admission. Since their aggressions grew with their helplessness, body belts and even hand and foot cuffs were additionally introduced. A truly perfect system of repression!

We live in the atomic age. We know of the atomic structure of all matter. But we have apparently realized little that we ourselves consist of atoms and their movements. Each of these atoms follows the back movements of attraction, repulsion, and orbiting, and these basic movements return on the level of the organs, the muscles, and the joints, and apparently also on the level of behavior in the way we react, how we are. It seems obvious that through the ubiquitously appearing atomic structure of matter and its energy, which moves everything, we are fundamentally connected with the whole. Perhaps this connection is only recognized when the liminality of the I-consciousness is loosened and the power of the will recedes, as is the case in psychosis. Many schizophrenics experience a much more direct connection to the whole than in their normal being or state.

"Central experience," I called this insight into the coherences of meaning in psychosis. Sigmund Freud identified something very similar in dreams: "Above all, there is a striking tendency to *compression,* an inclination to create new unities out of elements that we would certainly have kept separate in waking thought."[12] Is there really only a psychological mechanism at work, or is it that unifying driving force of life that Freud calls eros?

"The aim of [*Eros*] is to establish and maintain ever greater unities,"[13] Freud writes. This unifying force toward ever greater units is what we now experience in the striving for a unified Europe and in the collapse of dictatorships and their movement toward democracies. It is time that the psychiatric dictatorship cedes to a more democratic attitude. That would mean recognizing that not the NORM is the measure of all things but the human being with their needs. Then psychiatrists could work out an understanding of psychosis together with their patients, even learning from them.

12 Sigmund Freud, *An Outline of Psychoanalysis,* trans. Helena Ragg-Kirkby (London: Penguin, 2003), 196.

13 Ibid., 179.

11

The Glass Coffin

I saw Bethel again in 1977, twenty-four years after I was last here, and twenty-one years after my first experience in an institution. After twenty-one years I stood in front of the house where my fate had been decided, where I had had to bury my hopes for love, marriage, children, and a long-planned career, without being granted even the semblance of a choice. For years, the *Bethel Messenger* has been reporting successes in curative education, exercise, and occupational therapy, even with the most ill children in the "Patmos" House. It's been reporting the planned new building, "Siloah," on the forest's edge. Reporting more democracy in Bethel. I wonder if it would interest the doctors and nurses to learn how I came to understand my psychosis and cure myself. Though I don't remember a psychiatrist ever wanting to know how we experienced psychosis and what it meant for us.

It's Saturday and no doctor is available. The woman at the gate is barely willing to tell me anything, but eventually we get to talking as I reveal I was a patient here. I ask about the present procedures.

"Are group discussions held?"

"Yes," she says, "and medication, of course. And occupational therapy."

Walking by, I see a sign reading "Occupational Therapy" on the door to the room where I once built a big clay crib. A long wall hanging decorated with batik work and made by the patients hangs at the entrance. I like it a lot.

I want to see the ceramic wall the patients designed in the new semi-detached house, "Nazareth." The new "Place of Thanks" with its workshops is closed on the weekend, so this wall is all I get to see that's made by the patients. There are no more tours of Bethel. "We're not objects for people's entertainment," the patients said to justify their rejection. They were listened to — that too is new.

The semi-detached facility "Nazareth" is a long, spacious concrete building along Bethel's main street. Its modern architectural design immediately catches the eye. The new head administration building is covered in dark gold-colored metal panels. Usually, administration buildings are plain-colored to match the mundaneness of their function. Was the shimmering golden metal meant to show that the smelting works so important to Bodelschwingh were places of purification, and to continue the tradition of portraying Bethel as a city of God? The view is good, but I'm taken aback when I read that evening about the "Morija" house for mentally ill men in Raimund Hoghes's 1976 Bethel report, *Weakness as Strength:* "Waiting (for government subsidies) by the most severely ill, for example, must be done in repugnant sleeping quarters. Patients in this situation have, according to their doctors, an 'advantage' over those not so severely disabled: 'They can no longer perceive their surroundings.'"[1]

Humanitarian living conditions seem more important to me than a new administration building. I wonder if the doctors in 1936 believed that we or the "most severely ill" could no longer perceive our surroundings. Hardly, as, other than apathetic Little Marie, we were all too restless for that to be the case, too full of life. Luckily for us, there were no psychotropic drugs at the time, so we were able

1 Raimund Hoghes, *Schwäche als Stärke: Bethel ein Symbol und die Realität* (Neukirchen-Vluyn: Neukirchener Verlag, 1976), 46.

to keep ourselves fully conscious and retain our drive, even if we weren't allowed to act on it. The person who is respected less than an animal, who is denied even perception of their surroundings — "the Word of God" cannot give that person their human dignity back. When a person is subjected to medication and locked away for years, they can become as numb and indifferent as the patients in "Morija" were assumed to be.

I search in vain for the ceramic wall in the "Nazareth" building. It's in the closed assembly hall. Yes, I can go take a look; a young male nurse joins me. At the end of the long room there's an inlaid, colorfully glazed wall a little more than four meters wide. The prevailing color is a warm red. A scene from the New Testament is engraved in each roughly brick-sized tile, more refined and clearer than a "normal" person probably would have been able to produce. There are one-hundred-and-eighty-three biblical scenes on exactly the same number of tiles. Some stories are depicted in multiple images, others just in one. The individual elements of the picture stand in warm red in yellow, white, dark green, blue, or brown glaze. The color scheme and the composition of the plates were done by the couple who run the ceramic workshop. This original work was designed by a very young patient, seventeen at the time, as I read in a book the nurse gave me. About twenty other patients collaborated.

God is depicted as a white or yellow triangle with a halo. This symbol appears twice in the story of Abraham's test of faith. In his book, Johannes Busch reports on an argument among the patients:

> Hartmut Gnass first painted the symbol for God, the small triangle, on the sky, still half covered by a cloud. Consciously or unconsciously, he felt that God was far away from those inhuman events. However, a spontaneous discussion arose about this among the employees of the ceramics workshop. God, some said, was not

> distant or hidden from His people in the story of Abraham. Rather, one can find Him on Isaac and Abraham's paths, right at the point where obedience and sacrifice are expected from both of them.

"They talked about it for a long time," says Hartmut Gnass. "In the end, they even voted on where God should be found and therefore also drawn. And then he decided to engrave the symbol for God on the tile a second time. The first triangle, representing a distant, invisible, and incomprehensible God, could no longer be completely removed from the tile, and maybe it will remind the viewer of their own similar experiences with faith. But the second symbol, brightly and clearly etched exactly at the point where an almost-daring faith is expected of Abraham and Isaac, amounts to a personal confession: "Even when I can no longer see any connection between God and my life's path, it is precisely then that I would want to find him upon my path and be able to count on His being close to me."[2]

How could I not think of the instability I felt during my first episode, experiencing that which was incomprehensible and counter to all reason as divine guidance? Did that mean that religious experience was no longer being fought against during psychosis?

What a pity, I thought, that this work of art, born from the patients' experiences, is kept under lock and key and is only here for the twenty to twenty-five deacons and pastors who gather around the long table in this room. The patients worked on it for over a year. Wouldn't it strengthen their self-confidence if their work was available for all to see?

Later, in *Weakness as Strength,* I read about an experiment that the Swiss art action group Col began in Bethel in 1973: "Four weeks of work with patients, with people

2 Johannes Busch, quoted in Hoghes, *Schwäche als Stärke.*

who react differently than others, are themselves different. While painting together, making music, talking to each other, this otherness manifested itself in the following way, for example: The patients are less able to pretend than other people. Their personality emerges more strongly. They are more guileless.'" Another finding of the Col group: "In Bethel you could find several hundred people with significant creative abilities."[3]

Where will the new "Siloah" building be built? The *Bethel Messenger* had an article about the plan and asked for donations. The plan was for small living groups, each with a kitchen, so that the patients can prepare food themselves. On the way, I run into a patient and ask him for directions. He is already over fifty. In the fall, he'll move into the new "Emmaus" high-rise building for the elderly.

"It has become freer in Bethel," he says.

I'm walking beside the forest when I meet two patients of the house in front of "Morija." Their resignation in the face of being considered inferior is easy to hear in our conversation. It feels good to be able to reveal myself as one of them; here I can openly show what I otherwise have to hide. But how difficult it is to fight against their inferiority complexes! So much mental damage is left from an exclusively negative evaluation of anything they felt that deviated from the norm! I have to put so much work into convincing them of the value of our shared experiences!

"Actually, you're right," one of them finally says.

There is still nothing to be seen of "Siloah."

On Sunday, the next morning, I go to the Sarepta Chapel. Patients are organizing the service. A large harmonica choir in the sanctuary accompanies the singing instead of an organ. Then the patients play the parable of the workers in the vineyard. From the intense and genu-

3 Hoghes, *Schwäche als Stärke.*

ine patients' performance we feel what persuasive power the parables of Jesus must have had for his contemporaries.

This parable from the Kingdom of Heaven never seemed so real and vivid to me before. As everyone else makes their exit, I feel urged to thank the actors. I am so moved that I can hardly get the words out.

"Why aren't you playing in the bigger Zion Church?" I ask.

"The prophet counts for nothing in his fatherland," replies a little white-haired lady whom I had mistaken for a nurse.

"Are you a patient too?"

"I've been a patient at Bethel for sixty years. I'm seventy-two now."

The other guests are also moved by the performance of the patients, happening so close to them.

"Maybe we don't realize what the patients are until after they die," one nurse says.

Do we really have to have died first?

A few weeks later, I picked up *Bethel Workbook 3: Introduction to Psychiatry, Basic Psychiatric Questions, Psychopathological Systematics, Mental Abnormalities (Deviations).* Immediately I felt rage rise up in me, for what I read here differed only by a somewhat greater caution from what the somatists said decades ago about the "endogenous psychoses."[4] There is still talk of "incomprehensible and impalpable mental changes," from which "a deeper, precisely somatic event" is concluded.[5] With a viewpoint like that, Bethel's nurses could not be guided toward an understanding of psychosis as an awakening of the unconscious after mental conflicts and stresses, and

4 Winfried Rorarius, "Einführung in die Psychiatrie, Psychiatrische Grundfragen, Psychopathologische Systematik, Psychische Abnormalitäten (Abweichungen)," Bethel-Arbeitsheft 3 (Bethel bei Bielefeld: Verlagshandlung der Anstalt Bethel, 1973), 21.

5 Ibid.

without that understanding even the most selfless commitment could bring no real help.

The workbooks are read and probably accepted by many people working at Bethel, since the authors enjoy authority as experts. This upset me so much that I decided to conclude my report with a letter to the then head of Bethel. I would like to take him at his word, since he wrote that "the well-being of the patients is the highest law" in Bethel. I would like to ask him to make it possible for his patients to have a true and in-depth understanding of their psychosis and of themselves, and thus to experience the reality that "all things serve them for the best" — also and especially psychosis. But I keep mistyping and can hardly read my own writing. *Better to go into the garden and pull weeds,* I tell myself, and I do.

But then I experience something liberating. In the evening, a program comes on the radio: "Journey into Madness — Music, Poems, Pictures by Schizophrenics." The poems by schizophrenics from the psychiatric hospital in Klosterneuburg near Vienna impress me very much. The fact that their doctor, Leo Navratil, takes their experiences so seriously and considers them worthy of reflection seems to me like a promising approach. And the sympathetic comments of the show's author, Dieter Schlesag, fill me with relief and hope.

Afterward, standing in front of my bathtub where I'd been about to shower, I breathed deeply in and out, over and over. It was as if I was shedding the debasement I had experienced for over forty years. And then I burst into tears, liberating, cathartic tears. *You haven't felt this happy in a long time,* I thought afterward. The fact that I could feel included in the circle of these schizophrenics, that I knew my experiences were understood and accepted along with theirs, allowing me to completely identify with them — this let me breathe a deep sigh of relief that never seemed to end, as if my healing was now truly completed. They spoke of so many experiences that were familiar to me and that I hadn't been able to share with anyone before: the "rosette," the "central forms," the sensing of hidden complexes of meaning.

I reached again for Navratil's book *Schizophrenia and Art* and read some passages I had marked years ago, because his view of schizophrenia didn't match my experiences. Nor did it match the experiences of his patients from the radio program. "The schizophrenic experiences the total collapse of their ego and thus of the world,"[6] Navratil wrote. He means the functions of the ego such as reason and will. But what does he mean by the "collapse of the world?" And is this ego necessarily worth preserving? Or does it have to collapse in some cases so that further development becomes possible? I perceived my psychotic episodes as an expansion of my personality and as a sensitization, and the patients on the radio program seemed to feel similarly.

Does Leo Navratil also decide what the schizophrenic experiences by himself, rather than listening to them? He mentions a statement by Manfred Bleuler that the nature of schizophrenia remains "one of the greatest mysteries of our time." If this riddle can yield more insight, then it probably can only by way of the experiences of those affected.

Eighteen years had passed since I was cured, and now it's over thirty. The cure was complete; since then, I've had no further psychotic episode. I no longer needed one since I'd accepted the messages of my unconscious and integrated them into my life. My psychotic experiences have greatly enriched my life. But the shock at being debased and forcibly sterilized because of them has left me with deep wounds that continue to affect me to this day. In 1978, almost twenty years after I was cured, I had a nightmare about being in the asylum again.

6 Leo Navratil, *Schizophrenie und Kunst. Ein Beitrag zur Psychologie des Gestaltens* (Munich: Deutscher Taschenbuch Verlag, 1965), 15.

I was again in Bethel, but in a different building. My mother (she'd died over twenty years ago) and my sister had brought me. I don't know why they wanted to leave me here as a patient. It's early morning and I'm in bed. I'd just been typing up my account of my experiences in the asylum. In the dream, the red folder with the manuscript is lying next to me. A doctor in a white coat, tall and lean, enters the room and silently motions for me to come along. For a moment, I consider whether the report in the red folder can save me from an anesthetic injection. Surely the doctor would have to recognize from it that my psychosis is a spiritual affair that cannot be fixed with medication. *No,* I say to myself, *better he doesn't read it. He might try to stop it from being brought to light.* I follow the doctor through the corridors. Behind a door, I hear the desperate protest of a female patient. I'm so upset about being committed, which is completely incomprehensible to me, that I can only speak with difficulty and in a completely altered voice.

In the doctor's office. He doesn't say a word. I'm lying in a glass coffin with water flowing down its sides. *The water is a symbol from my unconscious,* I think. *But why am I lying in a glass coffin? So that the water of my unconscious doesn't reach me? Is that the purpose of psychiatric treatment?* Then I find myself facing the doctor again.

"Say something! Why am I here?"

He beckons me with his index finger, indicating that I should follow him.

"Stop waving your finger at me! Talk to me!" I manage with difficulty to say.

I follow him back through the halls. I still have this altered voice. I try to explain to him that it's not a symptom of illness, but because I'm so upset about being committed without any comprehensible reason. I can barely manage to speak. I'm back in the waiting room with my mother and sister. They look so kind and welcoming.

"I can't stay in this building! You'd better take me to the other Bethel building that I know!"

They are silent.

I wake up. Thank God it was a dream! And I can speak properly again. I say a few words out loud just to make sure. But what did the dream mean? Is this fear still ingrained so deep in me: once again being at the mercy of an anesthetic injection, unable to defend myself, being listened to by no one? Is that why I was in the coffin? Will we, who have experienced total powerlessness in the asylum, ever be able to get rid of this fear completely?

Since then, I have had in-depth conversations with other former patients. They, too, had undergone a changed perception of the world in a way very similar way to mine. Like me, they had also sensed otherwise hidden complexes of meaning and had valued their inner impulses, interpreting them as guidance.

"Through my psychosis I came to trust in God," one of them told me.

"The substance given to me by my experiences in psychosis sustains me to this day," said another.

When will psychiatrists finally have the empathy and understanding they need to accompany and gently guide patients along the path to a positive understanding of their own psychosis? When will they stop debasing and devaluing us?

Much has changed in recent decades. But mostly only on the surface. And some things have gotten worse. I was spared the permanent anesthesia and other damaging effects of psychotropic drugs. Nor did I experience being put in shackles, as Uwe Heitkamp reported in a program on April 9, 1986:

> I am lying in one of sixteen beds in the recovery ward. In this large glass cage, all the inmates are dozing off under the effects of psychotropic drugs. 5:30 am is wake-up time. Already at 7 o'clock they have to take

> pills. After that is breakfast. The use of violence is no exception here. And violence means being tied naked to the bed. In my ward with thirty-two people, two were treated like this every day.

"Concentration camps" is what one of the committed psychiatrists called such dreaded institutions, the ones with forced drug suppression, at the annual meeting of the German Society for Social Psychiatry in November 1985. He knew from his experience seeing the Bremen asylum, Kloster Blankenburg, repurposed into shared apartments, that it takes years of effort to enable such damaged long-term patients to lead self-reliant, humane lives again.

How many of those afflicted prefer suicide to such institutions? Some members of our self-help group tried to persuade a young woman who had recently come to us to be treated in a clinic. They drove her there that very evening. They sat with her in the car in front of the clinic for a long time, but she could not be persuaded to go in with them. From a previous stay at a clinic or institution, she knew what was likely to await her there. If she had found a true understanding of her inner problems during her previous stay in the clinic and not just had medical suppression, she would have been happy to take advantage of the help now. The group finally drove back without having achieved anything. The next day, the young woman jumped from a window. She jumped to her death.

Was it psychosis that destroyed that life? There are also healing forces at work in psychosis. For the person who is guided with understanding, it can mean a possibility of development and maturation, a chance for rebirth.

Bibliography

Arbeitskreis. "Geschichte Bethels," ed. *Lese-Texte zur Problemkreis "Eugenik, Sterilisation, Euthanasie."* Bethel bei Bielefeld: Verlagshandlung der Anstalt Bethel, 1983.

Bleuler, Eugen. *Dementia Praecox oder Gruppe der Schizophrenien.* Leipzig: Deuticke, 1911.

Bovet, Theodor. *Die Person: Ihre Krankheiten und Wandlungen.* Tübingen: Katzmann-Verlag, 1948.

Brandt, Wilhelm. *Friedrich von Bodelschwingh, 1877–1946.* Bethel bei Bielefeld: Verlagshandlung der Anstalt Bethel, 1949.

"Briefe." *Spiegel,* May 16, 1961. https://www.spiegel.de/politik/sterbehilfe-a-4b52ac67-0002-0001-0000-000043364022.

Die Zeit 1, February 21, 1946. https://www.zeit.de/1946/01/index.

Ebbinghaus, Angelika, Heidrun Kaupen-Haas, and Karl Heinz Roth. *Heilen und Vernichten im Mustergau Hamburg: Bevölkerungs- und Gesundheitspolitik im Dritten Reich.* Hamburg: Konkret-Literatur-Verlag, 1991.

Endres, Franz Carl. *Mystiek und Magie der Zahlen.* Zurich: Rascher, 1951.

Evangelische Kirche in Deutschland. *Evangelische Dokumente zur Ermordung der „unheilbar Kranken" unter der nationalsozialistischen Herrschaft in den Jahren 1939–1945.*

Edited by Hans Christoph von Hase. Stuttgart: Evangelisches Verlagswerk, 1964.
Fischer, Frank. *Irrenhäuser: Kranke klagen an*. Munich: Kurt Desch, 1969.
Flex, Walter. *Der Wanderer zwischen beiden Welten: Ein Kriegserlebnis*. Munich: Beck, 1916.
———. *The Wanderer between the Two Worlds: An Experience of War*. Translated by Brian Murdoch. London: Rott Publishing, 2014.
Freud, Sigmund. *An Outline of Psychoanalysis*. Translated by Helena Ragg-Kirkby. London: Penguin, 2003.
Gedat, Gustav Adolf. *Ein Christ erlebt die Probleme der Welt: Versuch einer volkstümlichen Einführung in das Weltgeschehen unserer Tage*. Stuttgart: J.F. Steinkopf, 1934.
Hoghes, Raimund. *Schwäche als Stärke: Bethel ein Symbol und die Realität*. Neukirchen-Vluyn: Neukirchener Verlag, 1976.
Jaffé, Aniela, ed. *Erinnerungen, Träume, Gedanken von C.G. Jung*. Zurich and Düsseldorf: Walter Verlag, 1993.
Jaspersen, Karsten. *Lehrbuch der Geistes- und Nervenkrankenpflege*. 7th ed. Bethel bei Bielefeld: Verlagshandlung der Anstalt Bethel, 1975.
Jung, Carl G. *Psychology of the Unconscious: A Study of the Transformations and Symbolisms of the Libido: A Contribution to the History of the Evolution of Thought*. Translated by Beatrice M. Hinkle. New York: Moffat, Yard and Company, 1916.
———. *Symbole der Wandlung: Analyse des Vorspiels zu einer Schizophrenie*. Edited by Jolande Jacobi. Zurich: Rascher Verlag, 1952.
———. *Wandlungen und Symbole der Libido: Beiträge zur Entwicklungsgeschichte des Denkens*. Leipzig and Vienna: Franz Deuticke, 1912.
Klee, Ernst. "Geldverschwendung an Schwachsinnige und Säufer." *Die Zeit* 18 (1986). https://www.zeit.de/1986/18/geldverschwendung-an-schwachsinnige-und-saeufer/komplettansicht.

Kretschmer, Ernst. *Medizinische Psychologie.* 3rd ed. Leipzig: Georg Thieme, 1926.

Leonhard, Karl. *Grundlagen der Psychiatrie.* Stuttgart: Ferdinand Enke, 1948.

Lienhard, Friedrich. *Thüringer Tagebüch.* Stuttgart: Verlag von Greiner und Pfeiffer, 1903.

Mitscherlich, Alexander, and Fred Mielke, eds. *Doctors of Infamy: The Story of the Nazi Medical Crimes.* Translated by Heinz Norden. New York: Henry Schuman, 1949

———. *Medizin ohne Menschlichkeit: Dokumente des Nürnberger Ärzteprozesses.* Frankfurt am Main: Fischer, 1960.

Mommsen, Helmut. *Der Gesundheits-Brockhaus: Volksbuch vom Menschen und der praktischen Heilkunde.* Wiesbaden: Brockhaus, 1951.

Navratil, Leo. *Schizophrenie und Kunst. Ein Beitrag zur Psychologie des Gestaltens.* Munich: Deutscher Taschenbuch Verlag, 1965.

Platen-Hallermund, Alice. *Die Tötung Geisteskranker in Deutschland.* Frankfurt am Main: Verlag der Frankfurter Hefte, 1948.

Rilke, Rainer Maria. *Selected Poems of Rainer Maria Rilke.* Translated by Robert Bly. New York: Harper and Row, 1981.

Rorarius, Winfried. "Einführung in die Psychiatrie, Psychiatrische Grundfragen, Psychopathologische Systematik, Psychische Abnormalitäten (Abweichungen)." Bethel-Arbeitsheft 3. Bethel bei Bielefeld: Verlagshandlung der Anstalt Bethel, 1973.

Siirala, Martti. *Die Schizophrenie des Einzelnen und der Allgemeinheit.* Göttingen: Vandenhoeck & Ruprecht, 1961.

Waggerl, Karl Heinrich. *Das Jahr des Herrn.* Wiesbaden: Insel-Verlag, 1933.

Made in the USA
Monee, IL
13 September 2026

62981965R00154